T0231184

Technology
in Social Work Education
and Curriculum:
The High Tech, High Touch
Social Work Educator

Technology in Social Work Education and Curriculum: The High Tech, High Touch Social Work Educator has been co-published simultaneously as *Journal of Teaching in Social Work,* Volume 25, Numbers 1/2 2005.

Technology in Social Work Education and Curriculum: The High Tech, High Touch Social Work Educator

Richard L. Beaulaurier, PhD, MSW
Martha Haffey, DSW, MSW, LCSW
Editors

Technology in Social Work Education and Curriculum: The High Tech, High Touch Social Work Educator has been co-published simultaneously as *Journal of Teaching in Social Work*, Volume 25, Numbers 1/2 2005.

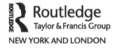

Routledge
Taylor & Francis Group
NEW YORK AND LONDON

First published by
The Haworth Press, Inc., 10 Alice Street, Binghamton, NY 13904-1580

This edition published 2013 by Routledge
711 Third Avenue, New York, NY 10017
2 Park Square, Milton Park, Abingdon, Oxon OX14 4RN

Technology in Social Work Education and Curriculum: The High Tech, High Touch Social Work Educator has been co-published simultaneously as *Journal of Teaching in Social Work,* Volume 25, Numbers 1/2 2005.

The development, preparation, and publication of this work has been undertaken with great care. However, the publisher, employees, editors, and agents of The Haworth Press and all imprints of The Haworth Press, Inc., including The Haworth Medical Press® and The Pharmaceutical Products Press®, are not responsible for any errors contained herein or for consequences that may ensue from use of materials or information contained in this work. Opinions expressed by the author(s) are not necessarily those of The Haworth Press, Inc. With regard to case studies, identities and circumstances of individuals discussed herein have been changed to protect confidentiality. Any resemblance to actual persons, living or dead, is entirely coincidental.

Cover design by Jennifer Gaska

Library of Congress Cataloging-in-Publication Data

Technology in social work education and curriculum: the high tech, high touch social work educator/ Richard L. Beaulaurier, Martha Haffey, editors.
     p. cm.
    "Co-published simultaneously as Journal of teaching in social work, volume 25, numbers 1/2 2005."
    Includes bibliographical references and index.
    ISBN-13: 978-0-7890-2961-4 (hc. : alk. paper)
    ISBN-10: 0-7890-2961-8 (hc. : alk. paper)
    ISBN-0-13: 978-0-7890-2962-1 (pbk. : alk. paper)
    ISBN-10: 0-7890-2962-6 (pbk. : alk. paper)
    1. Social work education–Technological innovations. 2. Educational innovations. 3. Internet in education. I Beaulaurier, Richard L. II. Haffey, Martha. III. Journal of teaching in social work.
HV11.T43 2005
361.3′071′1–dc22   2005006655

Technology in Social Work Education and Curriculum: The High Tech, High Touch Social Work Educator

CONTENTS

ABOUT THE EDITORS

Richard L. Beaulaurier, PhD, MSW, and **Martha Haffey, DSW, MSW, LCSW,** are Professors of Social Work at Florida International University, School of Social Work and Hunter College School of Social Work, respectively. Both authors have interest and expertise in the technology that enhances teaching and learning. In this book they hope to transmit this knowledge to their readers. As all the articles indicate, technology can enhance social work pedagogy when faculty have access to tools and frameworks to ease interpretation of techniques. This book highlights an important evolution in teaching.

Preface

There has been a dramatic increase in the use of computers and other forms of technology in social work education and in social work practice over the last several decades. The journal *Technology in the Human Services*, and its predecessor, *Computers in Human Services* have documented the remarkable rise in the use of technology by social workers. Many universities also see the use of emerging communications technologies as the key to reaching many non-traditional students who in distant locations and at unusual times. The Counsel on Social Work Education has even made introducing students to the latest developments in high technology an accreditation standard for schools of social work.

In spite of the rapid proliferation of technology, many social work faculty still wonder if the emphasis being placed on technology may have the unintended consequence of de-emphasizing social and interpersonal interactions–the "human" parts of the human services. Moreover, legitimate questions arise about how to bring technology into the educational experiences of students who are primarily there to learn about work with individuals and families in distress and the organizations and communities that serve them. Time and energy spent learning new technologies may, at times, feel like time away from these important activities.

Whatever reservations they have, however, few faculty and administrators in social work programs would dispute that they face considerable pressure to incorporate technology into their curricula, even if they do not feel completely familiar with the latest technologies, nor consider themselves sufficiently knowledgeable in their use. The situation

[Haworth co-indexing entry note]: "Preface." Beaulaurier, Richard L., and Martha Haffey. Co-published simultaneously in *Journal of Teaching in Social Work* (The Haworth Social Work Practice Press, an imprint of The Haworth Press, Inc.) Vol. 25, No. 1/2, 2005, pp. xix-xxiii; and: *Technology in Social Work Education and Curriculum: The High Tech, High Touch Social Work Educator* (ed: Richard L. Beaulaurier and Martha Haffey) The Haworth Social Work Practice Press, an imprint of The Haworth Press, Inc., 2005, pp. xiii-xvii. Single or multiple copies of this article are available for a fee from The Haworth Document Delivery Service [1-800-HAWORTH, 9:00 a.m. - 5:00 p.m. (EST). E-mail address: docdelivery@haworthpress.com].

is aggravated by the fact that technology manufacturers are well-known for exaggerating the benefits of their products, creating incompatibilities with existing or competing technologies, and for rapid obsolescence.

The authors in this volume have sought to address the concerns of social work educators in a variety of creative and interesting ways. Although differing approaches are taken, the common denominator is an emphasis on the use of technology to enhance and enrich learning about human relations, communities and organizations and how to improve them. The technology tail has not been allowed to wag the social work dog.

Moreover, the authors have endeavored to use plain language. Although the use and planning of technology will no doubt require new learning on the part of faculty, administrators, and students, the emphasis here is on technology that faculty can use with judicious investments of time and money, and on learning technology skills that are likely to be transferable even as hardware and software change over time.

Part I of this book contains five articles that examine innovative uses of technologies in areas of the curriculum that are not usually associated with digital technology. When the first digital computers began to appear they were seen largely as machines for making fast, accurate mathematical calculations. Perhaps for this reason, computer content in the curriculum has been most widespread in the areas of macro-practice (e.g., for budgeting, program planning and management information, and other management related functions) and for the quantitative aspects of research. More recently, information technologies have been making inroads into fieldwork, direct practice, social policy, and the *qualitative* aspects of research. These are the areas that are emphasized in the articles in Part I.

Social work was invested in distance education in the form of fieldwork long before universities began to make their push to embrace technological forms of distance education. More recently, advances in the same areas of technology that have made widespread use of distance education possible have been applied to the social work practicum. Birkenmaier and her colleagues develop models for using technology to improve the connection of widely distributed students and field instructors while at the same time creating stronger linkages between field experiences and the academic aspects of the curriculum.

MacFadden and colleagues challenge the common wisdom that technology has a deleterious effect on human relations. Their model suggests ways in which instructional technology can be used to emotionally engage students in the learning process. They draw examples from a course on cultural competency, itself an area not usually associated with on-line approaches to learning.

Other areas into which digital technology had made few inroads until recently are the teaching of social group work and qualitative research. Macgowan and Beaulaurier explore an approach to teaching about group practice using digital video and qualitative data analysis software. In so doing they demonstrate a flexible means of teaching students about group processes, while at the same time connecting direct practice to research. While the approach is directed toward the teaching of social group work, the same approach could be used in other areas of direct social work practice.

Few areas of social work have been as dramatically changed by technology as social policy. Moon and DeWeaver explore the way emerging communications technologies have revolutionized issue-oriented politics, and the new roles that these technologies play in advocacy. Roberts-DeGennaro and Clapp also examine the use of distance education technologies in policy education. Their empirical investigation of the technologies that students found most important and helpful in their learning, will be of interest both to social policy instructors and anyone else interested in adapting their coursework to distance education.

Articles in Part II examine the use of technology more globally in the classroom. Frey and Faul have developed an empirically grounded conceptual framework for incorporating web-assisted learning into traditional classroom settings. This should be of great assistance to the majority of social work faculty, who have yet to incorporate technology into their classrooms, but who are experiencing increasing pressure from their institutions and students to do so. Such faculty will also benefit by Sarnoff's article, which provides an overview of the benefits of web-based technologies that do not require learners and instructors to be present at the same time. In so doing, she explores one of the principal *advantages* that distance education has over more conventional approaches.

The chapter on interactive simulations by Seabury will be quite helpful to instructors who want to add an experiential component to the classroom experience, particularly in courses on direct practice. Reviewers felt that this article would aid instructors to visualize the potential for the use of such technologies in their own classroom.

More broadly, Beaulaurier and Radisch review the literature on computer aided instruction, with a particular eye toward CSWE guidelines requiring that technology content pervade the curriculum. The authors examine literature on the use of computers in every major area of the curriculum, as well as from four different approaches to the use of technology. The result is interesting with regard both to what areas have experienced a high degree of development of computer technology as well as areas that have received relatively little attention.

Part III steps back from the classroom to examine more global issues related to the use of digital technologies in social work education. The first article in this section, written by the editors, develops a model for planning the use and integration of computer technology in schools of social work and, more broadly, in social work curricula. The model takes into account factors that have been most challenging and perplexing to social work educators. These include the rapidly changing industry, development of new technologies, the obsolescence of old technologies, costs of developing and sustaining technology programs, and evaluating which technologies are most likely to be beneficial to faculty and students. The model develops an approach for cost-effective use and development of technology in an environment of constant change.

The second article in this section by Beaulaurier and Taylor addresses the age-old problem of getting help. Technology is rarely an end in itself for social workers, but rather a means to an end. As long as these technologies remain complex, it is likely that social workers will require the help of experts to set up, maintain and, importantly, to teach them how to use new software and hardware. This article, based on an empirical study, explores the behaviors of computer consultants noting that many of their behaviors actually seem to promote anxiety and have a deleterious effect on learning. This is instructive both for faculty and students seeking consultation, as well as for educators' monitoring of their own behavior.

In the final article of this section, Fitch takes a thoughtful look at the diffusion of technology in the human services. While the first article in this section develops a concrete model for technology planning, Fitch's article examines the incorporation of technology through the lens of diffusion of innovation theory. This theory guides understanding of when technology is likely to be most readily accepted and used, as well as when it is likely to be rejected. This thoughtful article complements the more concrete approaches taken in the other articles in Part III, as well as making an excellent capstone to the book.

Authors were asked to do seemingly paradoxical things: first, to make the writing accessible to readers who, while experts in their fields, were likely to be relative neophytes regarding technology; second, to write about approaches to the use of technology that are innovative and state of the art; finally, to write about *approaches* to the use of technology more than reviewing concrete exemplars of hardware or software.

Results exceeded our expectations. This work should appeal to a broad spectrum of social work educators and administrators, and should be of interest to novice and expert users of technology alike.

We have learned a great deal in the compilation editing this work and look forward to implementing what we have learned to benefit our own students and institutions. As one manuscript reminded us, social workers have embraced the latest technologies and scientific developments since the earliest days of the profession. We hope that you and your students will benefit from what we have learned in the development of this book as much as our own students have.

Richard L. Beaulaurier, PhD, MSW
School of Social Work
Florida International University, Miami

Martha Haffey, DSW, MSW, LCSW
School of Social Work
Hunter College, New York

PART I

Weaving a Web:
The Use of Internet Technology
in Field Education

Julie Birkenmaier
Stephen P. Wernet
Marla Berg-Weger
R. Jan Wilson
Rebecca Banks
Ralph Olliges
Timothy A. Delicath

Julie Birkenmaier, MSW, LCSW, Associate Clinical Professor, Stephen P. Wernet, PhD, Professor, Marla Berg-Weger, PhD, LCSW, Associate Professor, Director of Practicum, R. Jan Wilson, MSW, LCSW, Associate Clinical Professor, Rebecca Banks, MSW, LCSW, Associate Clinical Professor, are all affiliated with the Saint Louis University School of Social Service, St. Louis, MO. Ralph Olliges, PhD, is Assistant Professor, School of Education, Webster University. Timothy A. Delicath, PhD, is Director of Institutional Analysis and Assessment, Logan College of Chiropractic.

Address correspondence to: Julie Birkenmaier, MSW, LCSW, Saint Louis University School of Social Service, 3550 Lindell Boulevard, St. Louis, MO 63103 (E-mail: Birkenjm@slu.edu).

The evaluation component of this project was initially supported by Information Technology Services, Summer Fellowship Program, Saint Louis University.

This paper was presented at The Annual Program Meeting, Council of Social Work Education, March, 2001, Dallas, TX.

[Haworth co-indexing entry note]: "Weaving a Web: The Use of Internet Technology in Field Education." Birkenmaier, Julie et al. Co-published simultaneously in *Journal of Teaching in Social Work* (The Haworth Social Work Practice Press, an imprint of The Haworth Press, Inc.) Vol. 25, No. 1/2, 2005, pp. 3-19; and: *Technology in Social Work Education and Curriculum: The High Tech, High Touch Social Work Educator* (ed: Richard L. Beaulaurier, and Martha Haffey) The Haworth Social Work Practice Press, an imprint of The Haworth Press, Inc., 2005, pp. 3-19. Single or multiple copies of this article are available for a fee from The Haworth Document Delivery Service [1-800-HAWORTH, 9:00 a.m. - 5:00 p.m. (EST). E-mail address: docdelivery@haworthpress.com].

Available online at http://www.haworthpress.com/web/JTSW
Digital Object Identifier: 10.1300/J067v25n01_01

SUMMARY. The use of Internet technology in social work education is increasingly being debated. This paper describes applications using two technological tools to enhance one school's field education program. The development and current use of these computer-based strategies for use in the classroom-based Integrative Seminars, as a method to orient students to practicum and to offer an on-line Integrative Seminar, are discussed. Also described is the development of an additional project: the use of video conferencing technology to conduct virtual site visits. Key features, implications for the adoption of this technology in other programs, and student and faculty evaluation data are presented. *[Article copies available for a fee from The Haworth Document Delivery Service: 1-800-HAWORTH. E-mail address: <docdelivery@haworthpress.com> Website: <http://www.HaworthPress.com> © 2005 by The Haworth Press, Inc. All rights reserved.]*

KEYWORDS. Technology, social work education, field education

INTRODUCTION

Social work is a practice-based profession; therefore, considerable emphasis is placed on the field component of the curriculum. The field curriculum is designed to provide a supervised practice experience to apply the knowledge, skills, values, and ethics learned in the classroom (Council on Social Work Education, 1994). Field education is a central part of students' education and socialization and is increasingly suggested as the mechanism by which students gain exposure to contemporary forces impacting practice (Reisch & Jarman-Rohde, 2000; Strom-Gottfried, 1997).

The Office of Field Education and Faculty Field Liaisons are charged with implementing this crucial aspect of students' experiences. While models of field education vary in the type and purpose of contact between the agency and liaison and the role of the liaison (Fortune et al., 1995), liaison responsibilities generally include: (a) orienting students, field instructors and agencies to the roles, responsibilities, and expectations of the field program; (b) facilitating the integration of theory and practice; (c) teaching field seminars; (d) consulting with agencies regarding student learning; (e) monitoring students' progress in achieving learning goals and assessing professional development; (f) representing the program to agencies to foster dialogue between the two; (g) evaluating field instruction and support provided by the agency; and (h) evaluating student achievement while in practicum (Brownstein, Smith, & Faria, 1991; Fogel & Benson, 2000; Raphael & Rosenblum, 1987).

Field liaisons support both students and agencies in maximizing the learning experience of the student and provide a satisfactory supervision experience for the field instructor. Field instructors provide a crucial component of education for students, and field instructor satisfaction is vital to the success of the student's field education experience. Liaison availability and total number of contacts between the liaison and the field instructor are the best predictors of field instructor satisfaction with faculty field liaisons. Field faculty support, which may include emotional support, assistance with tasks, clear communication of expectations, and access to emerging information, is crucial to field instructors' satisfaction with field faculty (Bennett & Coe, 1998). Field education programs seek ways to provide the assistance, support, and communication needed for optimal field experiences for students and field instructors.

USE OF THE INTERNET TECHNOLOGY IN SOCIAL WORK EDUCATION

Citing possible negative effects on productivity, program development, and social relationships (Kreuger & Stretch, 2000), some social work educators caution against using Internet technology and distance learning in social work education. Despite the concern, the use of the Internet is being explored in most areas of social work curriculum. The Internet is routinely used in teaching course content to students in separate geographical locations. Distance learning is "a method of instruction involving two-way interactive televised transmissions between an instructor in one location and students elsewhere" (Thyer, Polk, & Gaudin, 1997, p. 363). Other non-interactive, Internet-based technology utilized in social work education involves Web pages, e-mail and other forms of communication to augment on-campus courses. Both distance learning and other Internet technology are used to teach in virtually all areas of undergraduate and graduate curricula (Siegel, Jennings, Conklin, & Napoletano Flynn, 1998), to include Human Behavior in the Social Environment (Siegel, Jennings, Conklin, & Napoletano Flynn, 1998), statistics and research (Harrington, 1999; Stocks & Freddolino, 1998), policy and macro practice (Fitzgerald & McNutt, 1999; Galambos & Neal, 1998) and social work practice skills (e.g., the use of interactive videodisk and computer-assisted instructional programs) (Coe & Elliott, 1999; Ezell, Nurius, & Balassone, 1991; McNutt, 2000; Maypole, 1991; Seabury & Maple, 1993). At least one program uses distance learning to teach all required undergraduate courses in rural areas (Haga & Heitkamp, 2000). Little discussion exists, however, on the organization of Internet-based field education strategies (Spencer & McDonald, 1998). The discussion and/or practice of Internet technology in field education is only beginning to emerge in the professional literature (Finn & Marson, 2001; Reisch & Jarman-Rohde, 2000; Siegel et al., 1998; Stofle, 1998).

Five factors, highlighted here, have prompted programs to consider the technology use in field education. Dramatic changes in the social service environment, to include managed care, have led to decreasing budgets and increasing expectations, thus, agencies have fewer resources and field instructors have less time for field supervision (Kolar, Patchner, Schutz, & Patchner, 2000). As a result, creative approaches to supervision are being suggested, such as shared student supervision, financial compensation for field instructors and increased use of University personnel (Birkenmaier, Rubio, & Berg-Weger, 2001; Bocage, Homonoff, & Riley, 1995; Jarman-Rohde, McFall, Kolar, & Strom, 1997; Raskin & Whiting Blome, 1998; Reisch & Jarman-Rohde, 2000; Rubio, Birkenmaier, & Berg-Weger, 2000; Strom-Gottfried, 1997). Consequently, practicum programs are seeking strategies to maximize supervision time and tools to compensate for decreased supervision from agencies. While field instructors place great emphasis on technology (Campbell & Queiro-Tajalli, 2000), most BSW and MSW programs are not using the Internet to facilitate field education (Finn & Marson, 2001).

Secondly, programs are searching for ways in which to recruit non-traditional, part-time students and students who commute long distances to attend school. Increasing the ease with which students can fulfill practicum and field seminar requirements through the use of technology can be an attractive feature to prospective students. Third, the use of distant sites for field education is increasing, posing challenging logistical and communication problems (Kilpatrick, Turner, & Holland, 1994). Fourth, students possess more sophisticated computer and Internet skills and want more efficient ways to obtain information about practicum, transmit practicum and seminar documents, and conduct site visits. Because computer technology is underutilized in the profession, researchers suggest that student computer literacy skills should be encouraged in social work education (Pardeck, Dotson, Ricketts,

McCully, & Lewis, 1995). Lastly, although the research is mixed, it does appear that computer-mediated communication can facilitate positive educational relationships (Gasker & Cascio, 2000; Mowrer, 1996; Savicki, Kelley, & Lingenfelter, 1996; Siegel et al., 1998). Therefore, the potential exists for the use of technology to further the educational goals of students in the field and maximize supervision and support without sacrificing positive educational relationships. Technology offers the opportunity to increase supervision and supportive resources for practicum students without increasing the burden on faculty, and increase the ease with which students can obtain field information and resources.

While the literature is replete with discussion and evaluation of technology in delivering curriculum (Coe & Elliott, 1999; Harrington, 1999; Johnson, 1999; Thyer et al., 1997; Thyer, Artelt, Markward, & Dozier, 1998), the scant literature available on the use of technology with field education has focused on individual field instruction (Stofle, 1998), the use of technology by field instructors (Campbell & Queiro-Tajalli, 2000), or distance field education programs (McFall & Freddolino, 2000). This paper describes one school's exploration of technology use in Field Integrative Seminars, in orienting advanced standing students to practicum, facilitating site visits and providing an on-line format for the Integrative Seminar. This paper will discuss three implemented projects (the use of Internet technology through the classroom-based Field Seminars, to provide an on-line Seminar format and to orient students to practicum) and one project currently under development (the use of web cams to facilitate site visits). Evaluation data regarding the implemented technology from students and faculty is provided.

INTEGRATION OF TECHNOLOGY AND FIELD EDUCATION– ONE SCHOOL'S EXPERIENCE: USE OF WebCT IN INTEGRATIVE SEMINARS

At the authors' Midwestern joint BSW and MSW program, the WebCT program has been integrated in the field program to enhance communication between students and between the instructor and students. The model of field education utilized at the university entails the use of specialized clinical faculty engaging in routine telephone contact with the agency and one in-person site visit for each semester. The MSW Integrative Seminars are conceptualized as a mechanism for the integration of classroom learning and practice experience gained in the practicum. The Seminar serves as a venue for further student-liaison communication and student support, to integrate classroom learning with the field experience as well as to learn more about social work practice in a variety of settings. Students are required to attend the Foundation seminar during their first practicum and a Concentration seminar during their second practicum. The Foundation Seminar is a zero-credit seminar designed to be part of the practicum experience. Students from each of the three concentrations are involved in the Seminar that meets for two hours three times/semester. In the Foundation Seminar, students debrief practice challenges and successes and integrate theory with practice by writing and presenting a case from their practicum experiences (Birkenmaier et al., 2001).

In contrast, the Concentration Seminar is a one-credit course completed concurrently with the first concentration-level practicum. Seminar activities also include debriefing, as well as exercises related to stress and diversity and the reenactment of a challenging case situation. Both Seminars are conceptualized as integral to the practicum experience.

Due to difficulty in meeting course objectives in the limited class time for the Seminars, the Practicum Faculty needed a tool to facilitate theory/practice integration and discussion of the experiences between class sessions. Additionally, faculty sought an easier mechanism to send documents to students, for students to send documents to each other and for documents to be made available to the entire class. The WebCT program was piloted as a tool for meeting these needs.

WebCT is an Internet program designed to enhance educational instruction. The software program offers the instructor the ability to create an interactive web site for the course. Tools also available to instructors and students through the program include: chat rooms; grade book; e-mail; test and quiz administration; and the ability to post documents to the entire class as well as to send documents to one another. The WebCT program offers confidentiality, as only students enrolled in the course have access to the course's web page.

Through a university technology fellowship program, Practicum Faculty received WebCT training via classroom instruction and individualized instruction and support. Practicum Faculty began using only several features in the first few semesters and later expanded the number of applications. Uses of the program currently include: (a) posting the Seminar syllabus and other documents; (b) on-line grade book; (c) links to on-line practicum forms and social work-related sites (e.g.,

NASW); (d) chat room to facilitate peer interaction; and (e) bulletin board to post discussion questions. Tools utilized at the beginning tended to be those that required the least knowledge about the program (i.e., posting of documents and grade book) and more sophisticated tools were used in subsequent semesters (i.e., chat rooms and links to other sites).

Two Examples

Of particular benefit is the ability of students to read documents ahead of time and use Seminar time to discuss, rather than present, case information. WebCT was used by several Faculty Liaisons to maximize the time available in Seminar. In the Foundation Seminar, a written and oral case presentation is required. The case presentation is designed to facilitate the integration of theory and practice. Using an outline that includes options for a micro, mezzo, or macro case, students select a challenging case from their practicum to present to other students for feedback. The case discussion familiarizes students with social work practice in other settings and facilitates the integration of theory and practice experiences. Prior to the use of WebCT, much of the time devoted to the cases was spent on the presentation of information about the case, leaving minimal time for discussion.

Discussion in the seminars has increased as students transmit their written case via WebCT to the instructor one week prior to the Seminar. The instructor can communicate with the student about the case, and once in the final format, upload the case for other students to read. All students, thus, have the opportunity to review the case and develop questions and comments. The presenting student reviews only the pertinent information before beginning a dialogue on the case using discussion questions he/she generated.

The use of the WebCT varies by instructor in the Concentration Seminars. Some instructors utilize WebCT only for posting documents and maintaining a grade book, while others interact with their students through the bulletin board option and provide concentration-specific links for student resources.

Evaluation

Using multiple strategies, evaluation of WebCT use in the Integrative Seminar has occurred. A focus group was conducted with four Faculty Liaisons and surveys and focus groups were completed with 121 Integrative Seminar students (Wernet et al., 2000). In general, students, and faculty reported positive experiences utilizing technology.

Student survey results demonstrated the importance of using technology to enhance communication between instructor and students, and among students. Faculty using WebCT to improve involvement through communication with and among students were more likely to increase students' satisfaction (B = .339, s.e. = .071, t = 4.799, p < .000) and this explained nearly half (49.8%) of the variance in students' satisfaction with the web-enhanced practicum seminar. Generally, students were moderately satisfied (X = 2.73, s.d. = .97) with the web-enhanced practicum seminar (Intercept: B = 3.488, s.e. = .862, t = 4.047, p < .000).

Developed through an iterative process, student focus groups were presented six questions. The questions focused on the student's experience with technology in the course, impact of technology on course progress, helpfulness of courseware tools, peer interaction and assistance and mastery of courseware. Students identified several positive aspects of utilizing WebCT in the seminar. First, the education experience is more convenient as the virtual learning environment is available 24-hours a day. Course information and course syllabi were readily available to students and could be accessed on demand. Secondly, the use of WebCt encouraged or forced students to become literate and competent in the use of computer technology, an important practice skill for contemporary practice. Third, the courseware empowered students by providing a sense of control over their time and, by extension, their lives as they could access and complete academic work at their most convenient times. Lastly, students felt that the courses were well-organized because of the use of technology and that faculty was more readily available to them through technology.

Challenges reported by students included: (a) students still experienced some access problems to both computers, in general (e.g., no computer at home, access to a "low end" machine only or prohibited at work), and the WebCT program, in particular. Specifically, student difficulties included inaccessibility due to port restrictions, bandwidth and/or network congestion problems, as well as occasional problems of compatibility between the browser software used by their Internet service provider (ISP) and the courseware (WebCT); and (b) students who struggle with computer and WebCT literacy reported frustration with time spent on technology issues versus on course substance. Students reported challenges with mastering the logic of sending attachments from within the courseware package, the need for greater ease of posting messages to the courseware bulletin board and frustration with the courseware's internal logic and structure for moving within and disconnecting from the courseware.

Faculty focus group feedback on the strengths include: the ability to provide more frequent and in-depth feedback to students; a more visible gradebook, enhanced theory and practice integration by students through online discussion; and greater flexibility for meeting submission deadlines. Additionally, students' work is more visible and available to others, which has encouraged students to turn in high quality work to be posted. Most students use computers and the Internet with relative ease, with only a small minority of students needing assistance with the technology. Faculty also noted that the usefulness of the technology must be clear before students can appreciate its role in the educational process.

ON-LINE INTEGRATIVE SEMINAR

While the use of distance learning in social work education is widespread, the use of Internet technology for Integrative Seminars has only recently begun to emerge. In response to increasing numbers of students commuting from a long distance and discussions of on-line seminars on a field listserve, the program recently launched an on-line version of the Foundation Integrative Seminar. The Seminar meets once in class at the beginning of the semester to orient students to the WebCT technology and to practicum, and the remainder of the course is held on-line. The course is held a synchronously using WebCT so that students can access course components at their convenience. Students have the same requirements as the in-class version of the course (described earlier) and use technology to discuss cases and their practicum experience. Students reflect on their practicum experiences and comment on other students' experiences by utilizing the bulletin board feature, write and send a case for uploading and discussion to the instructor, and comment on other students' cases using the bulletin board. Rather than diminish quality interaction, the instructor's experience is that the computer has enhanced practicum experience discussions and the integration of theory with practice, as the volume of feedback has increased to each student through the use of technology. To facilitate this, students are provided an explicit set of instructions regarding the quantity, quality and time frames for the various postings. Course evaluations are in the process of being adapted to include specific items about the on-line nature of the course.

USE OF WebCT–PRACTICUM ORIENTATION

After experience using the WebCT in Seminar for several semesters, the Faculty Field Liaisons progressed to experiment with the use of the WebCT as a supplement to the practicum orientation for advanced standing MSW students. Students typically receive advanced standing for practicum with a BSW degree from an accredited program. Unlike the non-advanced standing MSW students who were oriented during a Foundation course, this population was difficult to orient to practicum as they enrolled immediately in a variety of concentration courses and did not come together as a group. Due to anticipated scheduling problems with this population of students who are increasingly part-time and commuting from far distances, a mandatory, separate orientation was not a viable option. Faculty Field Liaisons were experiencing student non-compliance with practicum policies and procedures, many of which they felt were due to students' lack of knowledge.

To address this problem, an interactive orientation to practicum using the WebCT program was designed. Students were asked to read practicum orientation material uploaded onto the site, and encouraged to familiarize themselves with the practicum section of their student handbook. Students are required to complete and receive a passing score on an on-line quiz that tests their knowledge of practicum policies and procedures. The WebCT program scores the quiz and results are reported to the user and practicum secretary immediately. After students successfully complete the quiz, they may proceed with practicum planning for the next semester. Students who do not receive a passing grade must retake the quiz until a passing grade is achieved.

Evaluation

The experience with the orientation program has been positive. No formal evaluation has been completed, but Faculty Field Liaisons anecdotally report significantly fewer problems related to advanced standing students' knowledge of policies and procedures. Student feedback about the program has also been positive and the few problems that have surfaced with the technology have been easily remedied.

In sum, the WebCT program has proved to be a useful tool for both the field seminars and as a mechanism for orienting students to practicum. After such positive experiences with the WebCT program, the Liaisons are developing an additional project. The project involves the use of Web cams to conduct some site visits.

VIDEO-CONFERENCING FOR SITE VISITS

The program has an increasing number of students who commute from more than one hour away from the MSW program and want to complete practica in or near their home community. Field Faculty complete one site visit for each semester and find travel to be significantly increasing, straining their capacity to complete all field visits in a timely manner. Technology offers the possibility to assist in a more efficient and effective use of resources.

Video-conferencing involves the use of a small camera and microphone attached to two computers that allow the users to simultaneously see and talk with each other using the Internet in real-time communication. Although not widespread, the use of video-conferencing, or web cams, is beginning to be utilized for therapy (O'Neill, 2001). The use of cameras for site visits is a potential strategy to decrease the amount of travel without sacrificing instructor-student interaction and evaluation of the practicum experience. As no literature exists to guide the use of this equipment, the Liaisons are experimenting with various types of equipment and arrangements. Over the course of two years, the technology support for the University has assisted the field office in testing equipment, designing arrangements, increasing the capacity of the University and working with agencies willing to test the equipment and process. The equipment and arrangements are being tested and site visits are occurring at several sites with relatively sophisticated computer equipment in the metropolitan area. An essential part of the development of the project has been several pilot "virtual" site visits with agencies voluntarily recruited. For these pilot visits, the University provides equipment and technical support to the agencies.

Many problems have been encountered, including difficulty with the installation of the equipment in the agency and at the university, low-capacity agency computer equipment, lack of agency technical support, as well as faculty, student and field instructor initial unfamiliarity and discomfort with the technology. As with online therapy (O'Neill, 2001), the lack of appropriate computer bandwidth to allow quality video and audio transmission poses the greatest obstacle, as the small bandwidth causes a lag time for the transmission of pictures and words, which creates a significant decrease in the quality of the transmission and decreases the sense of a "real" interaction with the subjects in the field. These issues have lead to project delays until the bandwidth issue can be resolved. Although the project is delayed, the technology holds great promise for the future. Experts estimate that within only a few years, the technology needed for the project will be widespread (O'Neill, 2001), and the project can once again resume.

RECOMMENDATIONS FOR INTEGRATION OF TECHNOLOGY FOR FIELD EDUCATION

Several factors are proving vital to the success of the infusion of technology into the field education program. The review of helpful factors below serves as considerations and recommendations to programs considering the use of technology in field education. Such factors include:

Technological Infrastructure Within the Institution. Technological support and equipment from the University are vital to the success of these uses of technology. The University's commitment to the infusion of technology into the educational process resulted in a University technology fellowship for several projects. Individualized training and continual support provided by the fellowship during the design, implementation, and evaluation of all three projects have been instrumental. The social work program's commitment to purchasing the needed technology is critical.

Ability to Tailor the Use for Each Instructor. Although the initial use of the WebCT program was similar for each of the Liaisons, the features currently used in the Integrative Seminars vary widely. While some Liaisons use many features and/or offer an on-line Seminar, another Liaison offers only in-class Seminars and uses only a few tools of the WebCT program due to the changing needs of her field Seminar. Similarly, the use of web cams will be used to the extent that the Faculty Liaison is comfortable with and willing to use the technology.

Technology use is tailored to the teaching philosophy of the instructor. For example, an instructor who emphasizes the importance of supportive teacher-student relationships uses technology primarily to facilitate interaction and feedback. Another instructor who emphasizes the transmission of knowledge emphasizes the importance of lecture notes available on the WebCT (Lynn, 1999). The ability to customize technology to individual instructors is key to the success of the technology infusion and instructor satisfaction.

Investment in Technology and Education. The technology staff at the University was well-versed in the WebCT program when training the Liaisons. Faculty within the department who were using the program for instructional purposes have been instrumental in brainstorming ways in which the technology can be useful in field education. Additionally, the WebCT program was used in a variety of other courses within the social work program prior to the use in field education and many students were familiar with the educational advantages of the program. Based on student focus group findings, WebCT technical support must also be available to students as they become acquainted with the program and throughout their usage.

Adequate Access to and Support for the Technology. While access to computers was a concern at the outset, the university provides ample computer resources for students on campus. Students are advised that computers are also available at public libraries. Although some access issues linger, few students experience difficulty accessing computers. The issue of access to video-conferencing technology for practicum sites has been resolved during the pilot phase by limiting the number of sites and supplying the agencies with free equipment that they retain for future use. Due to cost constraints, the use of video conferencing for site visits is anticipated to be limited until future resources can be located to supply the technology or the equipment becomes standard for use in agencies.

Anticipation of Difficulties with Technology. The Liaisons plan for technological difficulties due to inadequate technological hardware, access issues and support at field placement agencies. For the WebCT program in the Seminars and the practicum orientation, faculty and staff are available to students for technological support. University technological support staff have been available for group training on the WebCT program, individualized instruction and problem-solving. Additionally, Liaisons create back-up procedures in case of technical difficulties. For example, if students have difficulty accessing the WebCT and are unable to contact the instructor, students are advised to send the paper through regular e-mail as an attachment. As stated, video conferencing technology is currently problematic, and Liaisons continue to conduct an in-person site visit or, if distance is an issue, conference telephone calling is used. When web cam technology becomes more widespread and less problematic, an in-person site visit will always be an option presented to the student and field instructor. Lastly, an in-class Integrative Seminar option will continue to be available to students as an alternative to the on-line version of the course.

Acceptance and Lead Time. When beginning to infuse technology in the program, planning for a lengthy planning and start-up stage and a gradual phasing in of technology is important. Potential barriers to infusing technology beyond technological considerations include acceptance and comfort with the technology by faculty, students, field instructors, and agencies. Building acceptance by students who are more reticent to attempt computer technology involves demonstrating the usefulness of the tools as well as providing support for technology challenges as they arise.

CONCLUSION

At the same time that the forecast for social work in the future suggests rapid and complex societal changes as a result of economic globalization, changing political climate, growing use of technology and demographic shifts in society, social work education is attempting to respond to the need for a closer alliance with field instructors. More frequent communication is designed to provide increased resources to more closely monitor students' field education progress (Reisch & Jarman-Rohde, 2000). While not without flaws and challenges, technology provides a variety of tools to enhance a quality field education experience for students. WebCT and video conferencing technology are two strategies that offer opportunities for meeting the needs of Field Faculty Liaisons, students and field instructors. Research on student satisfaction with the use of Internet technology is mixed, with some results showing students significantly favor live instruction to televised distance learning (Rooney & Bibus, 1995; Thyer et al., 1997; Thyer et al., 1998) and other research suggesting that Internet technology that supplements a course (such as a class e-mail project) enhances the educational experience (Gasker & Cascio, 2000). Further research is needed to demonstrate the effectiveness of distance learning and other Internet technology toward the practicum goals: student and field instructor satisfaction, the completion of student learning goals, increased communication and support for field instructors, and increased efficiency for practicum programs.

REFERENCES

Bennett, L., & Coe, S. (1998). Social work field instructor satisfaction with faculty field liaisons. *Journal of Social Work Education, 34*(3), 345-352.

Birkenmaier, J.M., Rubio, D.M., & Berg-Weger, M. (In press). Human service nonprofit agencies: Studying the impact of policy changes. *Journal of Social Work.*

Birkenmaier, J.M., Wilson, J., Berg-Weger, M., Banks, R., & Hartung, M. (In press). MSW Integrative Seminars. *The Journal of Teaching in Social Work.*

Bocage, M.D., Homonoff, E.E., & Riley, P.M. (1995). Measuring the impact of the fiscal crisis on human services agencies and social work training. *Social Work, 40*(5), 701-705.

Brownstein, C., Smith, H.Y., & Faria, G. (1991). The liaison role: A three phase study of the schools, the field, the faculty. In D. Schneck, B. Grossman, & U. Glassman,

Field education in social work: Contemporary issues and trends (pp. 237-248). Dubuque, IA: Kendall/Hunt.

Campbell, C., & Queiro-Tajalli, I. (2000). *Utilization of information technology by field instructors: Implications for curriculum development.* Paper presented at the 4th Annual Information Technologies for Social Work Education and Practice Conference. Charleston, SC, August, 2000.

Coe, J.A.R., & Elliott, D. (1999). An evaluation of teaching direct practice courses in a distance education program for rural settings. *Journal of Social Work Education, 35*(3), 353-365.

Council on Social Work Education (1994). *Handbook of accreditation standards and procedures.* Alexandria, VA: Author.

Ezell, M., Nurius, P.S., & Balassone, M.L. (1991). Preparing computer literate social workers: An integrative approach. *Journal of Teaching in Social Work, 5*(1), 81-99.

Finn, J., & Marson, S. (2001). The use of the world wide web by social work programs to facilitate field instruction. *Advances in Social Work.* In press.

Fitzgerald, E., & McNutt, J. (1999). Electronic advocacy in policy practice: A framework for teaching technologically based practice. *Journal of Social Work Education, 35*(3), 331-341.

Fogel, S.J., & Benson, M.V. (2000). Clarifying student competence in the agency setting: A model of practice for field liaisons. *Arete, 24*(2), 14-29.

Fortune, A.E., Miller, J., Rosenblum, A.F., Sanchez, B.S., Smith, C., & Reid, W.J. (1995). Further explorations of the liaison role: A view from the field. In G. Rogers (Ed.), *Social work field education: Views & vision* (pp. 273-293). Dubuque, IA: Kendall/Hunt.

Galambos, C., & Neal, C.E. (1998). Macro practice and policy in cyberspace: Teaching with computer simulation and the Internet at the baccalaureate level. *Computers in Human Services, 15*(2/3), 111-120.

Gasker, J.A., & Cascio, T. (2000). Computer-mediated interaction: A tool for facilitating the educational helping relationship. *The Journal of Baccalaureate Social Work, 5*(2), 145-159.

Haga, M., & Heitkamp, T. (2000). Bringing social work education to the prairie. *Journal of Social Work Education, 36*(2), 309-324.

Harrington, D. (1999). Teaching statistics: A comparison of traditional classroom and programmed instruction/distance learning approaches. *Journal of Social Work Education, 35*(3), 343-352.

Jarman-Rohde, L., McFall, J., Kolar, P., & Strom, G. (1997). The changing context of social work practice: Implications and recommendations for social work educators. *Journal of Social Work Education, 33*(1), 29-46.

Johnson, A.K. (1999). Globalization from below: Using the Internet to internationalize social work education. *Journal of Social Work Education, 35*(3), 377-393.

Kilpatrick, A.C., Turner, J.B., & Holland, T.P. (1994). Quality control in field education: Monitoring students' performance. *Journal of Teaching in Social Work, 9*(1/2), 107-120.

Kolar, P., Patchner, M.A., Schutz, Jr., W.V., & Patchner, L.S. (2000). Assessing the impact of managed care on field education in schools of social work. *Arete, 24*(2), 39-52.

Kreuger, L.W., & Stretch, J.J. (2000). How hypermodern technology in social work education bites back. *Journal of Social Work Educaton, 36*(1), 103-114.

Lynn, M. (1999). Selecting technology that suits your needs. *Center for Teaching Excellence, Saint Louis University, 1999 Newsletter.* Available from: http://www.slu.edu/collegges/gr/cte/newsletter1999/index.html

Maypole, D.E. (1991). Interactive videodiscs in social work education. *Social Work, 36*(3), 239-241.

McFall, J.P., & Freddolino, P. P. (2000). Quality and comparability in distance field education: Lessons learned from comparing three program sites. *Journal of Social Work Education, 36*(2), 293-307.

McNutt, J. (2000). Organizing cyberspace: Strategies for teaching about community practice and technology. *Journal of Community Practice, 7*(1), 95-109.

Mowrer, D.E. (1996). A content analysis of student/instructor communication via computer conferencing. *Higher Education, 32,* 217-241.

O'Neill, J.V. (2001). Webcams may transform online therapy. *NASW News, 46*(7), 4.

Pardeck, J.T., Dotson, B.M., Ricketts, A.K., McCully, K., & Lewis, A. (1995). A replication of a study exploring the utilization of computer technology by social workers. *The Clinical Supervisor, 13*(2), 127-140.

Raphael, F.B., & Rosenblum, A.F. (1987). An operational guide to the faculty field liaison role. *Social Casework, 68*(3), 156-63.

Raskin, M.S., & Whiting Blome, W. (1998). The impact of managed care on field instruction. *Journal of Social Work Education, 34*(3), 365-374.

Reisch, M., & Jarman-Rohde, L. (2000). The future of social work in the United States: Implications for field education. *Journal of Social Work Education, 36*(2), 201-214.

Rooney, R.H., & Bibus, A.A. (1995). Distance learning for child welfare work with involuntary clients: Process and evaluation. *Journal of Continuing Social Work Education, 6*(3), 23-28.

Rubio, D.M., Birkenmaier, J.M., & Berg-Weger, M. (2000). Social welfare policy changes and social work practice. *Advances in Social Work, 1*(2), 177-186.

Savicki, V., Kelley, M., & Lingenfelter, D. (1996). Gender, group composition and task type in small task groups using computer-mediated communication. *Computers in Human Behaviors, 12,* 549-565.

Seabury, B.A., & Maple, F.F. (1993). Using computers to teach practice skills. *Social Work, 38*(4), 430-439.

Siegel, E., Jennings, J.G., Conklin, J., & Napoletano Flynn, S.A. (1998). Distance learning in social work education: Results and implications of a national survey. *Journal of Social Work Education, 34*(10), 71-80.

Spencer, A., & McDonald, C. (1998). Omissions and commissions: An analysis of professional field education literature. *Australian Social Work, 51*(4), 9-18.

Stocks, J.T., & Freddolino, P. P. (1998). Evaluation of a World Wide Web-based graduate social work research methods course. *Computers in Human Services, 15*(2/3), 51-69.

Stofle, G.S. (1998). Online supervision for social workers. *The New Social Worker, 5*(4), 13-14, 23-24.

Strom-Gottfried, K. (1997). The implications of managed care for social work education. *Journal of Social Work Education, 33*(1), 7-18.

Thyer, B.A., Artelt, T., Markward, M.K., & Dozier, C.D. (1998). Evaluating distance learning in social work education: A replication study. *Journal of Social Work Education, 34*(2), 291-295.

Thyer, B.A., Polk, G., & Gaudin, J.G. (1997). Distance learning in social work education: A preliminary evaluation. *Journal of Social Work Education, 33*(2), 363-367.

Wernet, S.P., Berg-Weger, M., Birkenmaier, J.M., Wilson, R.J., Banks, R., Hartung, M., & Olliges, R. (2000). *The use of web-based technology in social work education.* Paper presented at the Council on Social Work Education Annual Program Meeting, New York, NY.

Achieving High Touch in High Tech:
A Constructivist, Emotionally-Oriented
Model of Web-Based Instruction

Robert J. MacFadden

Marilyn A. Herie

Sarah Maiter

Gary Dumbrill

SUMMARY. This paper explores how human service learners subjectively experience a web-based approach to learning. The course was a new iteration of an earlier course on enhancing cultural competency and involved a sample size of 72 participants. A course on cultural competency can be a difficult one to deliver via a web-based medium given the potentially powerful emotions and personal issues that it might elicit.

Robert J. MacFadden, MSW, PhD, Associate Professor, Marilyn A. Herie, MSW, PhD Candidate, and Gary Dumbrill, MSW, PhD Candidate, are affiliated with the Faculty of Social Work, University of Toronto, Toronto, Ontario, Canada. Sarah Maiter, MSW, PhD, is Assistant Professor, Faculty of Social Work, Wilfrid Laurier University, 75 University Avenue West, Aird Building, 4th Floor, Waterloo, Ontario, Canada N2L 3C5 (E-mail: smaiter@wlu.ca).

Address correspondence to: Robert J. MacFadden, MSW, PhD, Faculty of Social Work, University of Toronto, 246 Bloor Street W, Toronto, Ontario, Canada M5S 1A1 (E-mail: robert.macfadden@utoronto.ca).

[Haworth co-indexing entry note]: "Achieving High Touch in High Tech: A Constructivist, Emotionally-Oriented Model of Web-Based Instruction." MacFadden, Robert J. et al. Co-published simultaneously in *Journal of Teaching in Social Work* (The Haworth Social Work Practice Press, an imprint of The Haworth Press, Inc.) Vol. 25, No. 1/2, 2005, pp. 21-44; and: *Technology in Social Work Education and Curriculum: The High Tech, High Touch Social Work Educator* (ed: Richard L. Beaulaurier, and Martha Haffey) The Haworth Social Work Practice Press, an imprint of The Haworth Press, Inc., 2005, pp. 21-44. Single or multiple copies of this article are available for a fee from The Haworth Document Delivery Service [1-800-HAWORTH, 9:00 a.m. - 5:00 p.m. (EST). E-mail address: docdelivery@haworthpress.com].

21

Developing a climate of safety to encourage openness and sharing was an important goal for the course. The course was structured to include both individual and group level activities and assignments. In exploring the emotional topography of these learners, we employed an existing list of 23 sensations and examined these in the context of the learners' experiences including course satisfaction. *[Article copies available for a fee from The Haworth Document Delivery Service: 1-800-HAWORTH. E-mail address: <docdelivery@haworthpress.com> Website: <http://www.HaworthPress.com> © 2005 by The Haworth Press, Inc. All rights reserved.]*

KEYWORDS. Computer assisted learning, distance education, emotional responses research, direct practice, student satisfaction

Exploring the nature of the learners' subjective experiences within education rarely occurs, especially within an online course (MacFadden, Maiter, & Dumbrill, 2002). Except for learner satisfaction, internal variables such as emotions, are essentially ignored. Yet emotions have been termed the "On-Off Switch" for learning (Vail, 1994) and are correlated with variables such as effort, interest, and academic achievement (Pekrun, 1992). Given the increasing popularity of web-based instruction and the unique and innovative nature of this modality, it is important to examine how learners experience this approach to education, particularly the role of emotion in learning and in online learning. This article will explore this area and present a constructivist, emotionally-oriented model of online instruction that incorporates an emotional emphasis. Results from an experience using this model in a web-based course to enhance cultural competency will be presented, and the article will conclude with recommendations to assist in developing instruction that utilizes the participants' emotional experiences to facilitate learning.

EMOTIONS AND LEARNING

Sylwester (1994) remarks that emotion " . . . drives attention, which in turn drives learning and memory." Daniel Goleman (1997) notes that anxious, angry and depressed students don't take in information efficiently and do not learn well.

Priscilla Vail, in *Emotion: The On/Off Switch For Learning* (Vail, 2002), remarks that faced with frustration, despair, worry, sadness, or shame, children lose access to their memory, reasoning, and the capacity to make connections. Similarly, Pekrun (1992) observes that emotions may initiate, terminate or disrupt information and result in selective information processing.

In reviewing the role of emotions in instructional design, Astleitner (2000) indicates that emotions were originally ignored in favor of a heavy cognitive emphasis. Some designers believed that emotional goals were long-range and intangible while others thought that emotional education is the task of parents. Some believed introducing emotions might disturb important cognitive objectives.

The model of motivation and instruction by Keller (1983), and Keller and Kopp (1987) introduced emotional considerations in instruction. They believed that after a performance, a learner experiences an emotional response such as elation, pride, despair, or tranquility. Emotions were viewed as parts of the consequences of a learning process and they should be reinforced. While emotions were mentioned in this model, they were subordinated to motivation.

A later phase in instructional design was termed "affective or holistic education" and criticized the lack of emotional considerations in instruction. Emotions were considered "attitudes" which were primarily a way of being set toward or against an object or situation. Some theorists formulated several external conditions to facilitate emotional expression and development and these conditions were the first strategies to establish an emotional design of instruction (Martin & Briggs, 1986).

A newer approach advocates "emotional education" based on the concept of "emotional intelligence" (Goleman, 1997). This approach focuses on the development of emotional competencies such as being able to stay open to feelings, to reflectively engage or to detach emotionally, and to express emotions accurately. Emotions are the content of instruction. Resistance to this approach, in part, has occurred from instructors who are unwilling to reduce cognitive learning outcomes in favor of emotional ones. To overcome this objection, some instructors have integrated emotions into daily instruction through "hidden emotional education" (e.g., Adams, 1996) such as stories about emotional issues when teaching grammar.

More recently, an emphasis on "emotionally sound instruction" or instructional strategies to increase positive and decrease negative feelings during regular instruction (Taylor et al., 1994) has emerged. Feelings are viewed as the conscious recognitions of emotions (Greenberg & Snell, 1997). Influencing feelings through specific strategies are the main elements of the Emotional Design of Instruction (EDI) approach. The

FEASP-approach (Fear-Envy-Anger-Sympathy-Pleasure) by Astleitner (2000a, 2000b, 2001), reflects this EDI orientation and will be examined later.

Emotions and Online Learning

The importance of students' affective experience of online learning has not been well-recognized or articulated in the research literature. Traditional course evaluations typically assess perceived external variables such as content relevancy and clarity, instructor's knowledge and skill, and appropriateness of assignments (Wegerif, 1998). Although several studies report students' frustration with the technological demands of online courses (Dede, 1996; Feenberg, 1987; Perdue & Valentine, 2000), these frustrations are rarely examined in detail (Burge, 1994; Gregor & Cuskelly, 1994; Spitzer, 2001). Nevertheless, there is research to suggest that online courses need to consider the "emotional topography" (MacFadden, Maiter et al., 2002) of students' experiences (Brace-Govan & Clulow, 2000; Goldsworthy, 2000; Spitzer, 2001).

Hara and Kling (2000) note that most of the online learning literature is primarily promotional in nature with minimal reference to negative and personal experiences. For example, Carr-Chellman and Duchastel (2000) in an article titled "The Ideal Online Course" consider instructional design elements related to both course content and technology, but do not consider the emotional impact of these elements. Spitzer (2001) points out that the "high touch" is often de-emphasized in favor of the "high tech" in online distance learning, and argues that "until those enamored of the hardware and software acknowledge the importance of human intervention, the full promise [of Web-based distance learning] will not be realized" (p. 55). Similarly, Goldsworthy (2000) stresses the importance of affective dimensions to online learning. He notes that emotion and cognition are tightly interwoven, in that all cognition is, to some extent, socio-emotionally situated, and that affective elements need to be considered and incorporated in course planning and execution.

In his ethnographic evaluation of an online course for instructors, Wegerif (2000) found that individual success or failure seemed at least partially dependent on the extent to which course participants were able to cross a threshold from "feeling part of a community and feeling that one is outside that community looking in" (p. 38). Students on the "inside" perceived the course as warm and welcoming, while students on the "outside" viewed the online environment as a cold and unfriendly medium. Certainly, student experiences of trust and safety have been cited as central prerequisites in the creation of functional collaborative learning environments (Hughes et al., 2002), however more research is needed to understand the ways in which crossing the threshold from "outsider" to "insider" can be facilitated.

The consideration and analysis of students' affective experiences in web-based courses may be especially salient in subject areas that are explicitly designed to challenge underlying values, attitudes and beliefs. Van Soest and colleagues' (2000) evaluation of a Web-based discussion forum for a course on cultural diversity and societal oppression found the course content to be personally and professionally demanding for both students and faculty. The authors note that "the emotions that can be evoked in students places heightened pressure and responsibility on faculty to be responsive to process issues, including students' emotional needs" (p. 465). The combination of emotionally challenging course content and the unfamiliarity of the online learning medium for many students underlines the importance of theory and research into the affective dimensions of online learning.

Astleitner and Leutner (2000) have developed a model of "emotionally sound instruction" which consists of strategies to increase positive and decrease negative emotions within an instructional context. Designers must understand and use five basic categories of emotional conditions to produce emotionally sound instruction.

This FEASP model (Table 1) indicates that instructional designers should analyze emotional problems before and during instruction and respond accordingly. Strategies are suggested for each of the five emotional categories such as: ensure success, accept mistakes, create a relaxed situation, be critical but positive (for Fear reduction); use consistent and transparent methods of evaluation, inspire authenticity

TABLE 1. The FEASP Model

Feeling	Description
Fear	Negative feeling from judging a situation to be threatening
Envy	Negative feeling from the desire to either get something others have or not to lose something one already has
Anger	Negative feeling from being blocked from reaching a goal
Sympathy	Positive feeling or experience of feelings of other people who are in need of help
Pleasure	Positive feeling based on mastering a situation with deep devotion to an action

Based on Astleitner and Leutner (2000).

and openness, avoid unequal distribution of privileges among students, encourage comparisons with autobiographical standards (for Envy reduction); stimulate the control of anger, show flexible view of things, express anger constructively, don't show or accept violence (for Anger reduction); intensify relationships, encourage sensitive interactions, establish co- operative learning environment, implement peer helping (for Sympathy increase); and, enhance well-being, establish open learning opportunities, use humor, utilize play-like activities (for Pleasure increase).

Having had previous experience in constructing and facilitating a web-based course in enhancing cultural competency (MacFadden, Dumbrill, & Maiter, 2000), a new model of instruction was developed for this course which emphasizes the emotional dimensions of learning. While this model acknowledges the need to increase positive emotions and decrease negative emotions, it also recognizes that some frustration and disequilibrium is part of the challenge and process of learning.

THE CEO MODEL:
A CONSTRUCTIVISTIC,
EMOTIONALLY-ORIENTED MODEL
OF WEB-BASED INSTRUCTION

This model is based on a constructivistic approach to online learning that emphasizes the emotional dimensions in instruction and on utilizing these dimensions in learning. The authors based this approach on the available literature and earlier experience and research of the authors. Specifically, a constructivistic approach is learner-centered with less focus on detailed content and more emphasis on assisting the learner to formulate and reformulate ideas and meanings. These new understandings are based on challenging existing learning, exploring alternative models, and confirming and/or reformulating these understandings. Within a context of safety and trust, learners are challenged and must explicate their positions. Constructivism is designed to deepen understandings through challenging information, ordering, reordering, testing, and justifying the interpretations (Gold, 2001).

The emotional emphasis within this CEO model was incorporated, in part, to facilitate these constructivistic goals. Learning, and especially emotionally charged learning found in courses such as enhancing cultural competency, is strengthened when it occurs within an environment of safety combined with challenge. The CEO model is based on three learning stages which reflect the constructivist paradigm, enhanced by a focus on emotions.

The next section describes these three learning stages and then discusses the structure components of the CEO model.

LEARNING STAGES AND THE CEO MODEL

This section introduces the learning stages incorporated into the CEO model. The model differs from Astleitner and Leutner's (2000) approach which maximizes positive and minimises negative emotions. Certainly the technology used in online education should elicit positive emotions, given that frustration and discomfort with the mechanics of online education can never be helpful. With respect to educational content, however, emotional comfort may not always be pedagogically sound. Indeed, some theorists believe that the development of cognitive schema through which one understands the world only occurs through discomfort. Piaget (Bybee & Sund, 1982), for instance, believes that learners' perspectives and ways of understanding the world change when they are brought to a place of discomfort–when they recognize that the ways one understood events do not explain new information they are receiving and "disequilibrium" occurs. It is the discomfort of disequilibrium that generates new ways of understanding and stimulates paradigmatic shifts in thinking.

All learning is not at the paradigmatic level. For instance, learning that Columbus arrived on the coast of America in 1492 requires no shift in cognition. Yet recognizing that Columbus did not "discover" America because it already existed and the popular portrayal of his arrival as a "discovery" is an example of historic events being framed in a Eurocentric perspective, may require some learners to step outside of their established ways of thinking. Stepping outside established ways of thinking is essential in courses that deal with cultural competence and examine racism and other forms of oppression. Consequently, in this course focusing on students remaining comfortable and feeling pleasure was not pedagogically viable. Indeed, students elected to attend the course for the opportunity to examine the ways stereotypes, racism and other "isms" operate within society and perhaps within their own social work practice. To deliver the promised learning required learners to explore issues and engage in thinking that they might find uncomfortable. Rather than focusing on evoking positive emotions and minimizing negative ones, it was recognized that the course would evoke a range of both positive and negative emotions and the design focus was on how this mix of emotions might be managed in ways that would bring constructive learning outcomes. Strategies for managing these emotions involved a three-stage process shown in Table 2: establishing safety; providing challenges to participants' existing thought; providing new knowledge and facilitating new ways of thinking. These stages are not necessarily discrete and, in practice, may blend in with each other in a dynamic fashion.

Safety

Safety was established by developing non-blaming supportive "ground rules" and having participants review these when the course began. Participants were asked to adopt the principle that the course could only be a safe place for them, if they helped make it a safe place for others. It was everyone's responsibility to make the course a safe place. To achieve this, participants were asked to recognize that fellow participants have chosen to take part in the course because they were committed to addressing racism and other "isms." Participants, therefore, did not need to help change each other's "attitudes" toward diver-

TABLE 2. A Model for Online Education Focusing on Emotions and Paradigmatic Change

Stage	Purpose	Activity	Potential Feelings of Learners
1: Safety	To create a safe learning environment that facilitates risk taking and examining one's ways of thinking	Construct rules to foster free communication and ensure safety. Monitoring of communication to ensure compliance and safety	Safety, support & acceptance
2: Challenge	To provide the opportunity for participants to critically examine their knowledge and world views	Introduce exercises and processes that allow participants to step outside their existing ways of thinking	Disequilibrium, confusion, anxiety, frustration in a context of safety, support, & acceptance
3: New thinking	To create opportunities for engaging with new knowledge and gaining new ways of viewing the world	Introduce alternative knowledge and ways of viewing the world	"Ah ha!" moments leading to a new equilibrium, satisfaction, exhilaration

sity, but to assist each other to understand the implications for practice. Discussions were regularly reviewed by the facilitators to ensure learner safety was not being compromised and learners were encouraged to communicate privately (e.g., telephone, direct e-mail) if difficult issues arose.

Challenge

Challenging participants' thinking needed to occur in a non-threatening manner. Exercises were designed to critique one's thinking at a private, individual level and participants had the option of publicly debating the personal challenges that the course evoked. For instance, participants were asked to share their own culture with others by providing a link to a single website that reflected their culture. Participants were then asked to debate feelings this exercise evoked. Participants spoke of frustration and annoyance because they found it impossible for a single website to portray their culture and they felt discomfort that other participants might attempt to understand their culture based on a single source. With these emotions "switched on," participants were asked to consider the implications of this experience for the cross-cultural social work technique of Cultural Literacy. Cultural Literacy is a practice model that focuses on understanding the cultures of social work clients based on textbooks that catalogue the characteristics of various diverse cultures. For course participants who relied on cultural literacy methods in their own practice, disequilibrium occurred as they not only understood, but also experienced, the limits of catalogued definitions of culture. Empathy and sympathy for social work clients having their culture defined in this manner were also evoked.

New Thinking

Whenever disequilibrium occurred, it was important also to provide a means forward–to facilitate new ways of thinking. Consequently, each time information was introduced that might challenge participants' ways of working or thinking, new information and models were introduced to provide alternatives. In addition, each time a way of thinking or working was challenged, the strengths of that model were also reviewed. For instance, when the limitations of the Cultural Literacy model were identified, participants were also asked to work in groups to identify which parts of the model might still constructively inform their practice. This process ensured that only the weaknesses and not the strengths of practice models would be discarded by participants.

Of course, not all learners experienced disequilibrium when the course exercises caused them to experience the limitations of the Cultural Literacy approach. For some learners, these experiential exercises confirmed what they already knew. Such students helped others in the course group exercise processes and they were also able to clarify and reinforce their own learning that had taken place before the course.

Structure and the Online Model

Based on the model of learning stages presented above, a web-based course on enhancing cultural competency of human service providers was designed that would contain an emphasis on learner emotions. This was achieved through incorporating the following eight structural components:

1. *Rules about communication and Netiquette.* The course contained information on how to communicate online with other learners in a facilitative fashion. The issue of negative emotions and reactions that might be engendered in exploring the value-laden topic of culture was openly acknowledged and ground rules were set. The intent was to ensure that all views and learners would be "respected" and a safe environment created. Such safety would encourage learners to risk, challenge, and reformulate their ideas. The intent was to enhance the sympathy and pleasure emotions and decrease the fear, envy, and anger affect. Information about rules and communication was provided even before the course began to increase the sense of comfort and to establish common ways of communication.

2. *Autobiographical area.* A course area for informal biographies and pictures, to facilitate interpersonal connection and empathy was developed. This, again, reflects the need to increase "sympathy" emotions. The facilitators posted their biographies which included some personal information as well as pictures. This was especially important to combat the impersonal atmosphere that an online learning medium can foster. Students modeled their autobiographies on those posted by the facilitators by including personal information, thus creating a sense of connection among learners. Sharing autobiographical information assisted in creating a relaxed atmosphere and inspiring a sense of authenticity–both im-

portant for fear reduction and envy reduction (Astleitner & Leutner, 2000).

3. *Assignments.* For the first session, assignments were dedicated to mastering the technology, including being able to navigate within the course, send and receive e-mails and view online content, including web access. The intent here was to reduce the inevitable frustration that occurs when learners are exposed to new technology. Early frustration, especially, can lead to premature drop-out. The intent of this focus was to reduce anger and fear emotions and to encourage an early sense of mastery and pleasure.

4. *Interpersonal support.* Substantial interpersonal support was structured into the course. There were four personal contact sources (two facilitators, one project manager, and technical support persons from the e-campus provider) and three methods of communication: e-mail (personal and conference), telephone, and chat. Direct and timely support was essential. For most learners, this was the first experience with web-based learning and a variety of emotions from anger, frustration to excitement were common. These direct support persons were attempting to minimize fear, anger, and envy emotions and maximize the sympathy and pleasurable affects.

5. *A special group area.* Each small group had a special area within the course website where learners communicated with each other. A facilitator and recorder were selected by each group, and this was directed towards encouraging communication and dialogue and increasing the "sympathy" emotions. It also proved a safer place for discussion and debate about sensitive topics, as learners did not have to communicate with all other learners when exploring their ideas. They could communicate with members of their group before sending their ideas to the larger group. Messages posted to the larger group were sent by specific groups rather than a person from a group. Thus, any critique or disagreement of their ideas was not targeted at a person. These strategies helped to reduce fear and anger emotions.

6. *Individual and shared group assignments.* Individual assignments were designed in a graduated way to increase in complexity and ensure early successes and a sense of mastery. Additionally, the group assignments increased learner communication and understanding and were designed to enhance the "sympathy" emotions.

7. *Feedback mechanism.* During group discussions and after each group assignment, timely feedback was provided to learners. The

intent here was to increase the pleasure sensation by establishing a connection with the learners and by providing encouragement about the course work completed and a sense of mastery. During the discussions, students' names and a summary of their points were used frequently to reward and personalize the experience.

8. *Course content.* The content of the course was delivered through a variety of media technology including PowerPoint with real audio, text-based information, and web-based information. Case examples, humor, cartoons, and exercises with a fun element were used to deliver course content. The intent of the variety in presentation method and in the use of humor and other features was to reduce fear sensations and to increase pleasure sensations, respectively.

RESEARCH METHOD AND FINDINGS

The web-based course on enhancing the cultural competency of human service workers that employed the above model was conducted during the summer of 2001. This six-week course was evaluated as part of a research study at the Faculty of Social Work, University of Toronto, Canada. The course was non-credit, free of charge and included measures related to cultural competency and questions concerning the nature of the learners' experiences. This six-week, web-based course was structured to include both individual and small group level activities and assignments with weekly objectives, content, and assignments. Participants were asked to log on at least a few times each week to encourage group interaction and to maintain the focus on the topic of the current week. New content and assignments became available at the end of each week period to ensure that learners were focusing on the same material and issues at the same time. While this course emphasized interactivity, connection and working with others, it is important to recognize that more structured, individualized and non-collaborative web-based courses may result in different participant experiences.

Sample

The self-selected sample consisted of 72 individuals in human service professions with 18% holding a Bachelor of Social Work degree and 31% a Master of Social Work degree. There were a range of other professions reflected in the sample including nurses, psychologists, social service coordinators/managers, and teachers. Most of the participants were women (88%) with an age range from 26 to 60 (M = 41.88, SD = 9.11). The majority identified themselves as intermediate (63%) or advanced (28%) computer users. Fifteen percent described themselves as novice Internet users, while the majority were either intermediate (59%) or advanced (25%) Internet users. More than half (57%) resided in the greater Toronto area, under one-third (31%) came from elsewhere in Ontario and a small number (11%) from major U.S. cities. A majority (60%) practiced in an urban setting and the remainder (40%) worked in a rural/urban location.

Emotional Experience of the Course

In this study, online participants were asked how often they experienced a range of "sensations" such as excitement and frustration, and being active or feeling at risk. A list of sensations was developed by the authors based on the available literature and on the feedback from learners who had taken the course previously. There were 23 of these sensations listed and participants could choose from 0 (never) to 4 (always). These sensations can be characterized as essentially negative (e.g., isolation, inadequacy) or positive (e.g., satisfaction, comfort, safe) experiences. Of the 23 listed sensations, 11 can be identified as negative and 12 as positive. Positive and negative items were distributed in a balanced fashion throughout the list. Means scores were calculated for the 23 sensations and are presented in ranked form, from highest to lowest (see Table 3).

Within the above ranking, eight of the 10 highest-ranked sensations are positive while eight of the lowest-ranked are negative–suggesting that participants' online experience was predominantly positive. The negative sensation of frustration, however, is a significant experience and ranks high. The most frequent positive sensations relate to the experiences of safety, comfort, satisfaction, feeling competent, being active, skillful, and knowledgeable. For these participants, although frustrating at times, this online experience appeared to substantially contribute to their sense of competency which was a primary objective of the course. These sensations, however, address the learners' subjective sense of competency which may or may not correspond to their actual knowledge and skill.

TABLE 3. Means and Standard Deviations for Sensations by Rank Order

Sensation	M	SD	n
Safe*	3.05	.80	41
Satisfaction*	2.52	.80	44
Frustration	2.39	.87	44
Being active*	2.33	.89	43
Knowledgeable*	2.31	.72	42
Comfort*	2.31	.87	42
Competence*	2.30	.76	44
Isolation	2.23	1.14	44
Being skilled*	2.19	.77	42
Empowerment*	2.10	.92	41
Humor*	1.93	1.00	42
Being lost	1.89	.95	44
Excitement*	1.88	.93	43
Confusion	1.81	.93	43
Anxiety	1.67	.98	42
Connectedness with others*	1.65	.75	43
Passivity	1.64	1.06	42
Inadequacy	1.60	1.06	42
Exhilaration*	1.45	1.15	42
Dissatisfaction	1.50	.88	44
At risk	1.19	1.01	43
Powerlessness	1.10	1.10	42
Boredom	1.05	.92	43

*positive sensation

Isolation and the Need for Connectedness with Other Learners

In examining the qualitative data from the online postings and post-workshop interviews, two major thematic issues emerged. These overarching issues were *feelings of isolation* (or lack of connectedness) and *frustration with the technology*. Participants' experiences of isolation ranged from actively trying to engage the group, to those who did not engage with others due to technology or other barriers. An open-ended question on the course evaluation asked participants whether there were any emotional needs that were or were not addressed in this online course. The overwhelming theme in the responses to this question was the need to connect with others, to share, learn and understand. Twenty-nine participants responded to this question and 18 of these 29 made some comment relating to the issue of the need for more connectedness with other learners, more direct communication with others, and a need to reduce the isolation and to share one's experience with others. The need to be able to chat with others directly and in real-time was mentioned by six participants. This theme of disconnectedness that emerged through the online postings and qualitative interviews can be linked with the "safety" stage in the model discussed in the CEO model (previous section). Although a safe environment was facilitated by the instructors via the rules about communication and Netiquette and interpersonal support, many learners emphasized that connecting with peers was an essential component in feeling safe in discussing controversial and emotionally-charges issues.

Indeed, feelings of disconnectedness also colored the impressions of some participants about the suitability of the online environment in general for social interaction and community-building. Given that there is considerable research and practice experience supporting the effectiveness of online environments as sites of social and learning communities (Rheingold, 1993; Cook, 1995; Jones and Farquhar, 1997; Watson, 1997), it is important to further explore how interpersonal connectedness and collaboration can be better fostered in online environments.

Group Process, Time Issues, and Connectedness

Qualitative data suggest that the online participants in the cultural competence course struggled with group process issues related to the collaborative assignments. These issues seemed to stem from the asynchronous timing of the discussion, where group decision-making was hampered by participants logging on to the course at different times. In the traditional classroom, verbal dialogue takes place in the same place, at the same time, using well-established norms for collaboration and interaction. On the other hand, the online classroom is characterized by place and time independence, and computer-mediated communication (Grint, 1989; Barreau, Eslinger et al., 1993). Thus, group collaboration in the tasks of "planning, problem-solving, issue discussion, negotiation, conflict resolution, document preparation, and information sharing" can be rendered more complex and challenging for online learners (Barreau et al., 1993, p. 7). For example, groups in the cultural competence course spent considerable time and energy deciding who would post the weekly summary of the group's work to the main course conference area. This type of decision-making can be streamlined when individuals are communicating at the same time. The "challenge" stage in the CEO model attempted to engage learners in the critical examination of their underlying assumptions and worldviews through collaborative exercises and processes. However, the logistical difficulties of getting started on some of these group-based approaches seem partly due to the asynchronous nature of the discussion.

Davies (1989) points to the issue of "time coherence" in online conferences. He suggests that the unpredictable time lapse between sending and receiving messages in asynchronous environments makes group cohesiveness and task performance difficult to achieve. Although the online environment for the cultural competence course provided opportunities for information sharing and access 24 hours a day, this was done asynchronously. A number of subjects indicated that synchronous participation, whether in the form of text-based chat or a face-to-face component, would have decreased their feelings of isolation and promoted interpersonal connectedness. Structuring a face-to-face or synchronous component, (such as regularly scheduled chat times or a structured synchronous exercise) has been suggested in the literature, as well, as a solution to the problem of time coherence. As Davie and Wells (1991) note,

> Reciprocity in time means mutuality of experience, whether by sharing a joke or by knowing that classmates are simultaneously engaged in the same activity at the same time but in a different place. (p. 19)

Although not having to attend at fixed times was articulated as one of the major advantages of the online course by participants in this study as well as in other online learning experiences (Hiltz, 1997; Brace-Govan & Clulow, 2000; Wernet, Olliges et al., 2000; Cascio & Gasker, 2001; Valenta, Therriault et al., 2001), incorporating some elements of real-time interaction can be a helpful "ice-breaker," and is also more time efficient in completing certain group-based tasks. This could, in turn, better facilitate the "challenge" stage of the CEO teaching/learning model.

Participants in this course were also asked, "Were you aware of any patterns in your emotional experience of this online course?" An analysis of these opened-ended responses revealed frustration as the most predominant theme. Frustration was explicitly mentioned in 14 out of

32 open-ended comments to this question. Frustration resulted from factors such as: limited connectedness with others; limited participation by others; feeling lost; finding materials; technological problems and poor technical support; slowness of the computer; limited time available and feelings of guilt from not spending enough time on the course; and not being able to move ahead. Frustration was connected by the participants with withdrawing more, working individually, experiencing completion anxiety, and impeded performance. Problems with the technology, was identified as a significant theme. It was mentioned by six of the 10 respondents who offered comments. Three of these six respondents mentioned that the technological problems were overcome early: "The technology was not working out for me at first, but I got over that easily . . ." "Bit put off by the technology but was confident I could get beyond . . ."; "Difficulties with the technology were somewhat frustrating–especially right at the beginning . . .".

Role of the Facilitator

Reeves and Reeves (1997) suggest that the online experience is more constructivist for the learner with the instructor becoming a facilitator or "guide on the side" rather than a "sage on the stage." This fits with the CEO model's emphasis on "new thinking," where alternative knowledge and ways of viewing the world are introduced to learners. This approach to teaching and learning, however, must be more carefully examined and implemented as these new demands can be both exciting and challenging. Although online courses can be developed where facilitators are "guides on the side," they should also be prepared to act quickly and decisively in situations where it is evident that learners are becoming frustrated with a variety of situations which may range from the technology or a new pedagogical approach. Learners appreciate prompt feedback from facilitators as well as from other learners (Bonk & Cummings, 1998). Facilitators need to be careful not to forgo increasing interactivity in an effort to be less directional, as the amount of interactivity in distance education experiences is thought to contribute to perceived quality (Wagner, 1997). The themes of isolation and frustration were also issues for students in the online condition of Faux and Black-Hughes' (2000) course on social work history, and for graduate students in an online educational technology course (Hara & Kling, 2000). In their review of the literature on factors influencing the effectiveness of online education, Jung and Rha (2000) note that interpersonal interaction, social engagement, and knowledge of the technology are central to learning processes, satisfaction and achievement.

In the online cultural competence course, it was sometimes the case that the technology overshadowed the pedagogical goal of fostering new ways of thinking. In spite of 24-hour technical support, assistance from the course instructors, and help from one of the researchers (who functioned as a kind of unofficial "course coordinator"), many students continued to experience problems with accessing the course and navigating within it, or in using some of the course's features. One suggestion made by participants was to have the instructors check in with learners on an individual basis early on in the course. Although this would be more time-intensive at the beginning, this type of "outreach" function could help resolve technical difficulties early on, as well as uncover other barriers to participation. For example, one visually impaired participant in the online course required that other students post messages in 14-point font or larger. This individual had to repeat the request a number of times over the first three weeks before everyone "heard" the message. In the course of an individual check-in early on in the process, the instructors might have been informed of this student's requirement directly, and been able to provide assistance by setting font size as one of the posting guidelines for the group. This would also have given the participant more of a choice about whether to self-identify as visually impaired.

The above considerations and ideas emerging from the research provide some new insights into the structure and pedagogical enhancements that might have mitigated students' feelings of isolation and frustration as well as facilitated greater engagements with alternative perspectives, worldviews, and knowledge domains.

Understanding Non-Verbal Cues Online

Exploring sensations and emotions within an online environment is a difficult task (Hara & Kling, 2000). The meaning and context of the statements and accompanying emotions and sensations are not necessarily evident or clear. Face-to-face communication is highly complex and often relies on cues other than the words spoken. Indeed, Watzlawick (1967) indicates that we pay much more attention to the non-verbal, than to the verbal in spoken communication. What, then, happens to perceived meaning in text-based, online communication when these cues are lacking?

At a research debriefing after the course concluded, the facilitators of the course spoke of the "emotional magnification" that can occur when textual messages are devoid of their accompanying visual context. One has to imagine the learners' responses to challenging messages and therefore the facilitator may end up exaggerating the emotional impact on the learner. This was a particular problem in a course that included examining emotions within a cross-cultural practice context. The facilitators indicated that they were generally "softer" in the online course than a traditional course because they could not easily identify the emotional impact of their statements, challenges and critiques on the learners. One facilitator reported, " . . . So I think it's different from on-ground. I would push things more. Whereas, online I don't know if I'm pushing them away and so it's hard to do." In other words, the instructors felt somewhat constrained in challenging participants' thinking in the on-line environment because they did not have access to non-verbal cues that students were feeling safe.

This dynamic can also affect learner communication with online classmates. Some learners may be concerned about alienating others because their statements could be misread and the intended meaning is not as easily verified in an asynchronous environment. One common caution to new e-mail users is to avoid text-based humor because it is so easily misread.

Various online communities (e.g., see the URL *http://aol.about.com/library/101/bl-emoticons101.htm*) have attempted to overcome this online emotional vacuum through including an emoticon bar which is a user bar with a series of faces or text-based images reflecting specific emotions. The user clicks on the message-relevant emotion which is then imprinted in the text. Others are trying innovative ways to improve online communication. Emotional bracketing techniques (e.g., I'm nervous that you may not understand this technical term) have been developed within an e-therapy context to enrich the communication and to foster an online helping relationship (Collie, Mitchell, & Murphy, 2000).

CONCLUSION

The CEO Model of web-based instruction was able to provide the circumstances that promoted the needed feelings of safety and permitted learners to challenge, generate, critique, and construct new ideas. While the assignments promoted individual activity and group collaboration, changes need to be made in the model to promote more direct and timely communication to increase learners' sense of connection with each other. Such changes might include a preliminary face-to-face meeting of the class and regularly, weekly chat sessions.

The following are suggestions derived from our experiences, research, and the literature that are offered to enhance the emotional experience of learners. More research needs to be conducted to explore the impact of each of these processes and principles on the learning outcomes of web-based students.

- Emphasize the safety of learners.
- Set guidelines early to enhance learner safety, including "Netiquette" rules.
- Monitor discussions regularly to ensure learner safety.
- Act quickly if guidelines are not being followed.
- Normalize some disequilibrium and discomfort.
- Provide alterative knowledge and models and encourage new constructions by students.
- Monitor emotions and, *where appropriate*, minimize negative and maximize positive emotions.
- Encourage communication of emotions through emoticons, emotional bracketing, text, and other methods.
- Provide several sources of communication with other learners, facilitators, and technical support persons.
- Facilitators should connect regularly with individual learners, privately and through the course website.
- Connections should be made early between facilitators, technical support persons and learners, and problems related to technology should be addressed immediately and successfully within the first two weeks, in particular.
- Use biographical areas to encourage early connections among learners and facilitators.
- Use assignments to foster communication among learners and facilitators and to generate positive critique and new ideas.
- When responding to learners, summarize contributions and use names.
- Facilitators should explore several ways to understand how learners are experiencing course content. This could include private e-mails, small group and large group chats, anonymous on-line surveys, and systematically scanning course communication for emotional content.

REFERENCES

Adams, C. (1996). *Creating caring communities: What it takes to make real change in real schools.* ERIC-Paper No ED396415.

Astleitner, H. (2000a). Designing emotionally sound instruction: The FEASP approach. *Instructional Science*, 28, 169-198.

Astleitner, H., & Leutner, D. (2000b). Designing instructional technology from an emotional perspective. *Journal of Research on Computing in Education*, 32 *(4)*, 497-510.

Astleitner, H. (2001). Designing emotionally sound instruction. *Journal of Instructional Psychology*, 28, 209-219.

Barreau, D., Eslinger, C., McGoff, K., & Tonneson, C. (1993). *Group collaboration in the virtual classroom: An evaluation of collaborative learning in the virtual classroom of CMS 828S and the technology that supports it.* Retrieved June 1, 2002, from *http://www.hitl.washington. edu/research/knowledge_base/virtual-worlds/JOVE/index.html*

Bonk, C., & Cummings, J. (1998). A dozen recommendations for placing the student at the center of web-based learning. *Educational Media International*, 35 (2), 82-89.

Brace-Goven, J., & Clulow, V. (2000). Varying expectations of online students and the implications for teachers: Findings from a journal study. *Distance Education*, 21 (1), 118-135.

Brindel, M., & Levesque, L. (2000). Bridging the gap: Challenges and prescriptions for interactive distance education. *Journal of Management Education*, 24 (4), 445-457.

Brosnan, M. (1998). *Technophobia: The psychological impact of information technology.* London: Routledge.

Burge, E. J. (1994). Learning in computer conferenced contexts: The learners' perspective. *Journal of Distance Education*, 9 (1), 19-43.

Bybee, R. W., & Sund, R. B. (1982). *Piaget for educators* (2nd ed.). Columbus, OH: Charles Merrill.

Carr-Chellman, A., & Duchastel, P. (2000). The ideal online course. *British Journal of Educational Technology*, 31 (3), 229-241.

Cascio, T., & Gasker, J. (2001). Everyone has a shining side: Computer-mediated mentoring in social work education. *Journal of Social Work Education*, 37 (2), 283-293.

Collie, K. R., Mitchell, D., & Murphy, L. (2000). Skills for online counseling: Maximum impact at minimum bandwidth. In J. W. Bloom & G. R. Walz (Eds.), *Cybercounseling and cyberlearning: Strategies and resources for the millennium* (pp. 219-236). Alexandria, VA: American Counseling Association.

Cook, D. L. (1995). Community and computer-generated distance learning environments. *New Directions for Adult and Continuing Education*, 67, 33-39.

Davie, L. E., & Wells, R. (1991). Empowering the learner through computer-mediated communication. *American Journal of Distance Education*, 5 (1), 15-23.

Davies, D. (1989). Computer-supported cooperative learning: Interactive group technologies and distance learning systems. In R. Mason & A. Kaye (Eds.), *Mindweave: Communication, computers, and distance education* (pp. 228-231). Oxford: Pergamon Press.

Dede, C. (1996). Emerging technologies in distance education for business. *Journal of Education for Business*, 71 (4), 197-205.

Draves, W. A. (1999). *Teaching online*. Wisconsin: Learning Resources Network.

Faux, T., & Black-Hughes, C. (2000). A comparison of using the internet versus lectures to teach social work history. *Research on Social Work Practice*, 10 (4), 454-466.

Feenberg, A. (1987). Computer conferencing and the humanities. *Instructional Science*, 6 (2), 169-186.

Goleman, D. (1997). *Emotional intelligence*. New York: Bantam.

Gold, S. (2001). A constructivist approach to online training for online teachers. JALN 5 (1), June. Retrieved November 22, 2002 from the World Wide Web: *http://www. aln.org/alnweb/journal/Vol5_issue1/Gold/gold.htm*

Goldsworthy, R. (2000). Designing instruction for emotional intelligence. *Educational Technology*, 40 (5), 43-58.

Greenberg, M., & Snell, J. (1997). Brain development and emotional development: The role of teaching in organizing the frontal lobe. In P. Salovey & D. J. Sluyter, (Eds.), *Emotional development and emotional intelligence: Educational implications* (pp. 93-119). New York: Basic Books.

Gregor, S. D., & Cuskelly, E. (1994). Computer mediated communication in distance education. *Journal of Computer Assisted Learning*, 10, 168-181.

Grint, K. (1989). Accounting for failure: Participation and non-participation in CMC. In R. Mason & A. Kaye (Eds.), *Mindweave: Communication, computers, and distance education* (pp. 189-192). Oxford: Pergamon Press.

Hara, N., & Kling, R. (2000). Students' distress with a web-based distance education course. Retrieved September 27, 2000 from the World Wide Web: *http://www.slis. indiana.edu/CSI/wp00-01.html*

Hiltz, S. R. (1990). Evaluating the virtual classroom, In L. M. Harasim (Ed.), *Online education: Perspectives on a new domain* (pp. 133-183). New York: Praeger.

Hiltz, S. R. (1994). *The virtual classroom: Learning without limits via computer networks*. Norwood, NJ: Ablex Publishing.

Hiltz, S. R. (1997). Impacts of college-level courses via Asynchronous Learning Networks: Some preliminary results. *Journal of Asynchronous Learning Networks*, 1 (2), 1-19.

Huff, M., & Edwards, S. (1999). *Using technology in a social work diversity course*. Retrieved September 27, 2000 from the World Wide Web: *http://www.cc.utah.edu/ ~jy1415/techconf/Docs/papers/Huff.htm*

Hughes, S. C., Wickersham, L., Ryan-Jones, L., & Smith, S. A. (2002). Overcoming social and psychological barriers to effective online collaboration. *Educational Technology and Society*, 5 (1), 1-10.

Jones, M. G., & Farquhar, J. D. (1997). User interface design for Web-based instruction. In B. H. Khan (Ed.), *Web-based instruction*, (pp. 239-244). Englewood Cliffs, NJ: Educational Technology Publications, Inc.

Jung, I., & Rha, I. (2000). Effectiveness and cost-effectiveness of online education: A review of the literature. *Educational Technology*, 40 (4), 57-60.

Keller, J. M. (1983). Motivational design of instruction. In C. M. Reigeluth (Ed.), *Instructional design: Theories and models* (pp. 386-434). Hillsdale, NJ: Erlbaum.

Keller, J., & Kopp, T. (1987). An application of the ARCS model of motivational design. In C. M. Reigeluth (Ed.), *Instructional theories in action* (pp. 289-320). Hillsdale, NJ: Erlbaum.

Khan, B. (1997) (Ed.). *Web-based instruction.* Englewood-Cliffs, NJ: Educational Technology Publications, Inc.

Kirkup, G. (1999). Technophobia: The psychological impact of information technology. [Review]. *Computers & Education,* 323, 279-280.

Lockee, B. B., Burton, J. K., & Cross, L. H. (1999). No comparison: Distance education finds a new use for "no significant difference." *ETR & D,* 47 (3), 33-42.

MacFadden, R. J., Maiter, S., & Dumbrill, G. (2002). High tech and high touch: The human face of online education. In H. Resnick & P. Anderson (Eds.), *Innovations in technology and human services: Practice and education.* New York: The Haworth Press, Inc.

MacFadden, R. J. Dumbrill, G., & Maiter, S. (2000). Web-based education in a graduate faculty of social work: Crossing the new frontier. *New Technology in the Human Services,* Vol. 13, No. 2.

Martin, B., & Briggs, L. (1986). *The affective and cognitive domains: Integration for instruction and research.* Englewood Cliffs, NJ: Educational Technology Publications.

McIsaac, M., & Gunawardena, C. (1996). Distance education. In D. Johnassen (Ed.), *Handbook of research for educational communications and technology* (pp. 15-38). New York: Praeger.

Newlin, M., Wang, A., & Kosarzyski, M. (1998). *Who succeeds in Web-courses?* Paper presented at the EDUCOM, Orlando, FL.

Noble, D. F. (1999). Digital diploma mills, Part IV, Rehearsal for the revolution. Retrieved September 27, 2000, from the World Wide Web: *http://www-rcf.usc.edu/~ics/ed/ddm4.html*

Pekrun, R. (1992). The impact of emotions on learning and achievement: Towards a theory of cognitive/motivational mediators. *Applied Psychology,* 41: 359-376.

Perdue, K. T., & Valentine, T. (2000). Deterrents to participation in Web-based continuing professional education. *American Journal of Distance Education,* 14 (1), 7-26.

Reeves, T., & Reeves, P. (1997). *Effective dimensions of interactive learning on the World Wide Web.* In B. Khan (Ed.), *Web-based instruction* (pp. 59-66). Englewood Cliffs, NJ: Educational Technology Publications, Inc.

Rheingold, H. (1993). *Virtual communities: Homesteading on the electronic frontier.* Don Mills, Ontario: Addison-Wesley.

Salanik, G. R., & Pfeffer, J. (1978). A social information processing approach to job attitudes and task design. *Administrative Science Quarterly,* 23, 224-253.

Spitzer, D. R. (2001). Don't forget the high touch with the high tech in distance learning. *Educational Technology,* 41 (2), 51-55.

Stock, J. T., & Freddolino, P. (2000). Enhancing computer-mediated teaching through interactivity: The second iteration of a World Wide Web-based graduate social work course. *Research on Social Work Practice,* 10 (4), 505-518.

Sylwester, R. (1994). How emotions affect learning. *Educational Leadership,* 52 (2). Retrieved November 22, 2002 from *http://www.ascd.org/readingroom/edlead/9410/sylwester.html*

Taylor, S., Aspinwall, L., & Guiliano, T. (1994). Emotions as psychological achievements. In S. H. M. van Goozen, N.E. van de Poll, & J. A. Sergeant (Eds.), *Emotions: Essays on emotion theory* (pp. 219-239). Hillsdale, NJ: Erlbaum.

Vail, P. (1994). *Emotion: The on/off switch for learning.* Rosemont, NJ: Modern Learning Press.

Vail, P. (2002). Emotion: The on/off switch for learning. Retrieved November 22, 2002 from: *http://www.schwablearning.org/pdfs/expert_vail.pdf*

Valenta, A., Therriault, D., Dieter, M., & Mrtek, R. (2001). Identifying student attitudes and learning styles in distance education. *Journal of Asynchronous Learning Networks,* 5 (2), 111-127.

Van Soest, D., Canon, R., & Grant, D. (2000). Using an interactive Website to educate about cultural diversity and societal oppression. *Journal of Social Work Education,* 36 (3), 463.

Wagner, E. (1997). Interactivity: From agents to outcomes. In T. Cyrs (Ed.), *Teaching and learning at a distance: What it takes to effectively design, deliver, and evaluate programs* (pp. 19-26). San Fransisco: Jossey-Bass.

Watson, N. (1997). Why we argue about virtual community: A case study of the Phish.net fan community. In S. G. Jones (Ed.), *Identity and communication in cybersociety* (pp. 102-132). London: Sage Publications.

Watzlawick, P. (1967). *Pragmatics of human communication.* New York: W.W. Norton.

Wegerif, R. (1998). The social dimension of asynchronous learning networks. *Journal of Asynchronous Learning Networks,* 2 (1), 34-49.

Wernet, S. P., Olliges, R. H., & Delicath, T. A. (2000). Postcourse evaluations of WebCT (Web course tools) classes by social work students. *Research on Social Work Practice,* 10 (4), 487-504.

Using Qualitative Data Analysis Software in Teaching About Group Work Practice

Mark J. Macgowan
Richard L. Beaulaurier

SUMMARY. Courses on social group work have traditionally relied on in-class role plays to teach group work skills. The most common technological aid in such courses has been analog videotape. In recent years new technologies have emerged that allow the instructor to customize and tailor didactic experiences to individual classes and individual learners. This article discusses the use of technologies such as digital video combined with computer aided qualitative data analysis software (CAQDAS). Two examples illustrate the use of Atlas.ti, a popular CAQDAS program, for advancing group work education. The use of data analysis software in group work courses gives students concrete examples and experiences in using research in group work practice. While

Mark J. Macgowan, PhD, LCSW, Associate Professor, and Richard L. Beaulaurier, MSW, PhD, Associate Professor, are affiliated with the School of Social Work, Florida International University, Miami, FL.

Address correspondence to: Richard L. Beaulaurier, School of Social Work, Florida International University, 11200 Southwest 8th Street, HLS II 364B, Miami, FL 33199 (E-mail: beau@fiu.edu).

[Haworth co-indexing entry note]: "Using Qualitative Data Analysis Software in Teaching About Group Work Practice." Macgowan, Mark J., and Richard L. Beaulaurier. Co-published simultaneously in *Journal of Teaching in Social Work* (The Haworth Social Work Practice Press, an imprint of The Haworth Press, Inc.) Vol. 25, No. 1/2, 2005, pp. 45-56; and: *Technology in Social Work Education and Curriculum: The High Tech, High Touch Social Work Educator* (ed: Richard L. Beaulaurier, and Martha Haffey) The Haworth Social Work Practice Press, an imprint of The Haworth Press, Inc., 2005, pp. 45-56. Single or multiple copies of this article are available for a fee from The Haworth Document Delivery Service [1-800-HAWORTH, 9:00 a.m. - 5:00 p.m. (EST). E-mail address: docdelivery@haworthpress.com].

this article discusses the use of such technologies in teaching group work, the approach could be adapted for use in other direct practice courses and in direct practice settings. *[Article copies available for a fee from The Haworth Document Delivery Service: 1-800-HAWORTH. E-mail address: <docdelivery@haworthpress.com> Website: <http://www.HaworthPress.com>* © 2005 by The Haworth Press, Inc. All rights reserved.]

KEYWORDS. CAQDAS, qualitative research, group process, group therapy, social work education, computer assisted teaching, distance education

Social group work educators in academic and field settings have traditionally utilized a range of methods for teaching group work skills. Some of the traditional written tools for teaching social group work include process recording, group work log, and group analysis (Getzel, Kurland, & Salmon, 1987; Graybeal & Ruff, 1995; Kurland & Salmon, 1998, pp. 205-206; Wayne & Cohen, 2001). In addition, most group work educational programs require students to observe experienced group workers leading groups and, more importantly, to lead or co-lead groups under supervision (Association for Specialists in Group Work, 2000; Shapiro, Peltz, & Bernadett-Shapiro, 1998; Wayne & Cohen, 2001; Yalom, 1995). Most would agree that the passive method of observing groups should be ancillary to active work with groups (Wayne & Cohen, 2001).

The most important technological innovation in the teaching of social group work has come with the advent of inexpensive videotaping equipment. In a survey of 212 faculty in BSW and MSW programs concerning teaching about group work, almost all (92%) of group work educators found videotapes to be very useful (Birnbaum & Wayne, 2000). In an early edition of his book, Yalom noted that videotapes held "considerable potential benefit for the teaching, practice, and understanding of group therapy" (Yalom, 1975, p. 437). Tapes are valuable in that they "provide access to more subtle elements of interaction such as tone of voice, the rhythm of the interactions, and body language" (Wayne & Cohen, 2001, p. 63). As Yalom has noted, "valuable teaching sessions which clearly illustrate some basic principles of therapy may be stored and teaching videotape library created" (Yalom, 1995, p. 426).

As useful as standard videotaping methods have been, the survey noted above revealed that the most frequent faculty recommendation (25%) was for the development of new and better teaching materials (Birnbaum & Wayne, 2000). Advances in technology allow the further development of visual media for teaching group work. New and increasingly affordable digital technology allows the instructor to create interactive experiences that can be manipulated by instructors and learners. This allows for a more experiential learning approach, commonly cited as a requirement in the education of group workers (Conyne, Wilson, & Ward, 1997; Wayne & Cohen, 2001).

HOW DIGITAL VIDEO AND QUALITATIVE SOFTWARE ADVANCE PREVIOUS TECHNOLOGY

The use of computer technology has become more frequent in teaching social work practice (e.g., Engen, Finken, Luschei, & Kenney, 1994; Falk, Shepard, Campbell, & Maypole, 1992; Maple, 1994; Maypole, 1991; Poulin & Walter, 1990; Seabury & Maple, 1993; Wodarski, Bricout, & Smokowski, 1996). In some cases these technologies are similar to current digital video technologies such as large videodiscs or programs resident on computers with limited distribution (Goldberg-Wood & Middleman, 1987; Maple, 1994; Maypole, 1991). More recently technologies have emerged that include examples of practice skills on portable compact disks that now accompany text or workbooks about individual (Haney & Leibsohn, 1999) and group practice (Haney & Leibsohn, 2001). While these technologies are considerably more autodidactic than their predecessors, none of these approaches have allowed students and faculty to directly manipulate video, and in particular, video of their own behaviors. However, the current generation of digital video technology, in conjunction with developments in data analysis software, makes this possible and practical.

Digital Video

As the technology has advanced, digital video recordings have come to have virtually the same advantages as analog recordings, with some additional advantages. Although the initial quality of digital recordings was inferior to analog, current technologies rival or exceed the standards of analog recordings. The principal advantage of digital recordings is the potential for interfacing with other digital technologies, especially the personal computer and the Internet.

As hard drives have gotten larger, video compression formats have gotten better and processing speeds have gotten faster, the ordinary desktop or even notebook computer has acquired the capability to play high quality video. Moreover, the average new desktop computer gives users access to complex editing techniques far beyond the reach of most analog video users who do not have access to sophisticated editing equipment.

Digital video can be copied with no loss of quality to the recording. Digital video can be stored cheaply and, importantly, can be transmitted easily over the Internet. This gives digital video a distinct advantage over other approaches for use in distance education. Moreover, there is an increase in use of electronic classrooms designed for the presentation of computerized images. Thus, digital images can be presented on the same hardware as other presentation formats such as PowerPoint, web-browsers, spreadsheets, and other specialized computer applications.

Qualitative Data Analysis Software

Since the 1980s a variety of tools have been developed to assist qualitative researchers in the analysis of data (Fisher, 1997). These packages are often referred to as computer aided qualitative data analysis software, or CAQDAS. Most CAQDAS packages have been developed primarily for the analysis of text (Drisko, 1998; Irion, 2002; Weitzman, 1999). In the past, qualitative researchers have often had to transcribe video and audio recordings to analyze them. The advantage of directly analyzing digital video recordings over text is that a more nuanced and holistic representation of the situation under study may be obtained (Irion, 2002; Koch & Zumbach, 2002; Weitzman, 1999). For this reason, some CAQDAS programs have added features that allow them to analyze other sources of qualitative data including still images, audio, and video (Irion, 2002; Weitzman, 1999).

Probably the two best known and most full featured qualitative data analysis software packages are NUD*IST-NVivo and Atlas.ti (Barry, 1998; Drisko, 1998). While both programs have incorporated capability for dealing with digital video, at this writing NUD*IST-NVivo allows links to video clips, but does not allow video segments to be coded directly. By contrast, Atlas.ti allows for the coding of entire video files. Although there are several other programs that are more specialized for qualitative analysis of video data (Koch & Zumbach, 2002), the authors chose to use Atlas.ti for the examples in this paper due its flexibility and popularity.

This paper will not attempt to discuss all of the uses of CAQDAS. Discussion will be restricted to features relevant to the pedagogical use that we will be putting the software. However, in order to understand the benefits of using CAQDAS, a short discussion of the basics of Atlas.ti and some fundamental principles of qualitative data analysis will be instructive.

Atlas.ti, like most CAQDAS packages, began development as a program for analyzing text. Thus, all computer files that constitute the raw data for Atlas.ti are called "primary documents." Although called "documents," these data can be in the form of text files, digital audio recordings, digital still images, or digital video. Data files are grouped into projects called HUs (Hermeneutic Units) by Atlas.ti. An instructor might, for example, create an HU for each new class. Each video associated with the class would be a primary document organized under the HU for the class.

The latest version of Atlas.ti (4.2 as of this writing) has the ability to read a variety of digital video formats including Mpeg, AVI, and QuickTime. Once a digital video segment has been entered into an HU as a primary document, the user can begin the process of transforming the data into smaller, meaningful segments (Figure 1). In the general parlance of qualitative research this is the process of "coding." Coding is a semiotic process where the whole of the video segment is broken down into smaller units of meaning, referred to as "quotations" by Atlas.ti.

A quotation is a sub-segment of video, and is tied to the time-code of the primary document file. If we are examining a video file of 30 minutes in length, the user might create a quotation beginning at 1 minute, 20 seconds and ending at 1 minute, 40 seconds. The user can create as many quotations as are needed, and quotations can be as long or as short as the user wishes to make them.

Once a quotation has been created, the user can add other objects, the two most important of which are "codes" and "memos." Codes are "named concepts" that can be assigned to other quotations. For example, the user may wish to create a code for "purpose statement." Once a code has been created, it can be assigned to any quotation in which there is an incidence of a purpose statement. Thus any named concept (code) can have one or more incidences (quotations) assigned to it. The creation of codes for major concepts makes it possible to arrange and show a variety of examples of concepts, from one or many video recordings,

FIGURE 1. Coding Process Using Atlas.ti: Relationship Between Objects

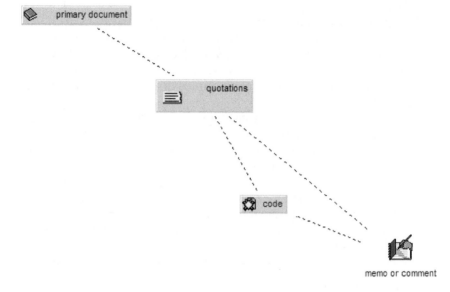

at the click of a button. Moreover, examples of concepts can come from sessions that the instructor has saved as exemplars, or from recordings of students' own sessions.

User-added commentaries can be added to any Atlas.ti object. In the literature on qualitative data analysis, such commentaries are known as "theoretical memos" (Strauss, 1987). Atlas.ti has two different strategies for creating theoretical memos. Atlas.ti contains an object called a "memo," which is a commentary that can be attached to any object in Atlas.ti. Atlas.ti also allows the user to attach a "comment" to any of its objects which is also a commentary. There are differences between memos and comments, but for our purposes, the differences between them are unimportant. In the interest of simplicity, the authors have elected to use only the "comments" feature of Atlas.ti as a way of adding commentaries to documents, quotations, and codes.

APPLICATIONS FOR GROUP WORK EDUCATION

Two examples illustrate the use of Atlas.ti for group work education. The first relates to the observation of experts in which educators identify skills or processes coded for display in video segments. The second involves students coding and commenting on their own work. The examples demonstrate the educational value of this coding process using two core competencies for group work practice derived from the Association for the Advancement of Social Work with Group's Standards for Social Work Practice with Groups (Association for the Advancement of Social Work with Groups, 2000); namely, encouraging member-to-member interaction, and establishing the group's purpose statement.

Observation of Experts

An important task in group work is to foster connections between members (Association for the Advancement of Social Work with Groups, 2000, Standards IIIC and IIID). One strategy that helps to foster member-to-member communication is to deflect comments of members directed to the worker, directing them instead to the rest of the group. Jacobs and colleagues suggest that,

> The leader should explain to the members that she/he would not be looking at them all the time when they speak because she/he needs to scan the room and that your scanning should serve as a clue for them to address themselves to the other members. (Jacobs, Masson, & Harvill, 1998, p. 105)

The instructor can create videos of actual groups and then code the video using Atlas.ti to mark behaviors such as "scanning the group with one's eyes while a group member is speaking." Group work educators could provide a set of examples for student reference. These examples could then be easily and cheaply distributed to students on CDs, DVDs or via the Internet. In addition to examples created by the professor, exemplars using student models could be created. This latter approach is preferable, since learning is generally enhanced when the models are similar to the learner (Bandura, 1986). Moreover, this approach lends itself to asynchronous, auto-didactic approaches to learning that have several advantages over conventional classroom approaches (Sarnoff, in this volume).

Student Coding and Commenting on Their Own Work

A more active approach to learning group leadership skills is for students to code and comment on their own work in an adaptation of conventional process recording methods. This process has the benefit of not only having students critically review their own group work skills, but also allows students using Atlas.ti to embed process comments directly in the video. Once coded, the students are able to quickly flip through sections of the video where they have problems, and compare their performance to that of exemplars provided by the instructor. This approach also allows the instructor to view sections of video with student comments attached, thus giving the instructor considerable insight into the student's critical skills. Such an approach allows the instructor to give more sharply focused feedback to students.

Process recordings using videotapes have several advantages over paper and pencil approaches. These include more accurate recall and the ability to be replayed for later review, allowing educators and students to examine the subtleties of group interaction (Graybeal & Ruff, 1995). However, written recordings have advantages in that they allow students to make comments about their intentions, thoughts about what went right or wrong, and what might be done to make improvements. By giving users the ability to combine text commentaries with video recordings, Atlas.ti can combine the advantages of both approaches. The advantage of this approach is highlighted in the following example.

A critical task at the outset of group is to clearly introduce and clarify the purpose of the group (Standard, IIIA, Association for the Advancement of Social Work with Groups, 2000). Workers who have mastered the skill succinctly introduce "their vision for the group, their hopes for group accomplishments, and their reasons for, and the agency's interests in, bringing the group members together" (Kurland & Salmon, 1998, p. 47). The skill associated with setting the purpose of the group has been coded in Atlas as "purpose statement" (Figure 2).

In the example in Figure 2, the process recording has been linked to a video recording of the beginning of a group. A code has been created for the skill: namely, making a purpose statement. The appropriate quotation has been highlighted and shown in its own window. Within the quotation window the specific sub-segment of video associated with the student's purpose statement has been highlighted. The comment box in the quotation window contains the student's answer to the following questions posed by the instructor, which are part of the process recording format: (a) what was the skill or technique? (b) What was the empirical or theoretical basis for the technique (with citation)? (c) What was the outcome of the technique–did it go as planned? (d) What would you say or do differently next time? At the bottom of the screen is a window showing all of the quotations that have been coded to "purpose state-

FIGURE 2. Atlas.ti Video Coding Screen[1]

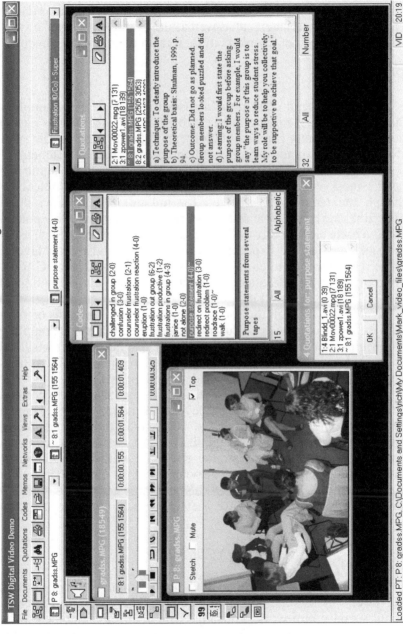

ment" even if they are in other videos. This feature allows the student to view their purpose statement as well as the example provided by the instructor, and/or other members of their team in group assignments.

Other Uses

There are several other possible uses for Atlas.ti. For example, Atlas.ti is capable of mixing media through hyperlinks. In this case, the user can assign any combination of text, video, or other media such as still images or sound recordings to an HU as primary documents. For the sake of brevity, the authors utilize a strategy that uses some of Atlas.ti's most basic functions, and which can be learned quickly. Although the techniques involved for linking mixed media through hyperlinks are more advanced, the stategy offers considerable potential, and is a more elegant way of linking lengthy text to video. Such uses are probably beyond the expectations for bachelor and master level students. However, instructors with advanced knowledge of CAQDAS programs may be interested in creating multimedia presentations that link text, video, and still images using hyperlinks.

In addition, through the use of more advanced functions of Atlas.ti such as "focused networks," users can graphically display complex relationships and links between concepts. This could have considerable value in showing the relationships theorized in group work writings, by grounding them in the reality of videotaped groups.

A complete exploration of advanced features such as hyperlinking and focused networks would be beyond the scope of this discussion. The two examples described above require only the basic features and understandings of Atlas.ti and qualitative data analysis; the coding and commenting techniques illustrated above are well within the reach of most instructors and students. The potential of the more advanced functions of Atlas.ti and other CAQDAS programs are more easily understood once basic functions have been mastered.

CONCLUSIONS

This paper has demonstrated a relatively simple method for exploiting the enormous potential of modern CAQDAS programs for teaching about social group work. Educators can adapt this approach to other modalities such as work with individuals or families. Such software is particularly helpful in cases where populations are culturally different, pre-lingual, or have other characteristics that make *seeing* and *hearing* important elements of understanding and treating.

Atlas.ti has considerable potential for helping students to bridge the gap between research and practice. In using the software to learn about groups, students also learn the fundamentals of qualitative data analysis, and the practical application of research techniques. Students who master these techniques have the potential of continuing to apply it to their practice in ways that have yet to be conceptualized. While CAQDAS software has been coming into wide recognition as indispensable to researchers with qualitative data, clearly the potential for the use of such programs has barely been tapped by educators and clinicians.

NOTE

1. Figure 2 was created with an older version of Atlas.ti (ver. #4.2). A newer, much improved version of Atlas.ti is now available. Used with permission.

REFERENCES

Association for Specialists in Group Work (2000). *Professional standards for the training of group workers.* Retrieved June 22, 2003, from: http://www.asgw.org/training_standards.htm

Association for the Advancement of Social Work with Groups (2000). *Standards for social work practice with groups.* Retrieved June 23, 2003, from: http://www.aaswg. org/

Bandura, A. (1986). *Social foundations of thought and action: A social cognitive theory.* Englewood Cliffs, NJ: Prentice-Hall.

Barry, C. A. (1998). Choosing qualitative data analysis software: Atlas/ti and Nudist compared. *Sociological Research Online, 3*(3).

Birnbaum, M. L., & Wayne, J. (2000). Group work in foundation generalist education: The necessity for curriculum change. *Journal of Social Work Education, 36*(2), 347-356.

Conyne, R. K., Wilson, F. R., & Ward, D. E. (1997). *Comprehensive group work: What it means and how to teach it.* Alexandria, VA: American Counseling Association.

Drisko, J. W. (1998). Using qualitative data analysis software. *Computers in Human Services, 15*(1), 1-19.

Engen, H. B., Finken, L. J., Luschei, N. S., & Kenney, D. (1994). Counseling simulations: An interactive videodisc approach. *Computers in Human Services, 11*(3/4), 283-298.

Falk, D. R., Shepard, M. F., Campbell, J. A., & Maypole, D. E. (1992). Current and potential applications of interactive videodiscs in social work. *Journal of Teaching in Social Work, 6*(1), 117-136.

Fisher, M. (1997). *Qualitative computing*. Adershot, UK: Ashgate.

Getzel, G., Kurland, R., & Salmon, R. (1987). Teaching and learning the practice of social group work: Four curriculum tools. In J. Lassner, K. Powell, & E. Finnegan (Eds.), *Social group work: Competence and values in practice* (pp. 35-50). New York: The Haworth Press, Inc.

Goldberg-Wood, G., & Middleman, R. (1987). Interviewing skills for the human services: Learner's workbook. Park Forest, IL: OUT ST Software.

Graybeal, C. T., & Ruff, E. (1995). Process recording: It's more than you think. *Journal of Social Work Education, 31*(2), 169-181.

Haney, J. H., & Leibsohn, J. (1999). *Basic counseling responses: A multimedia learning system for the helping professions*. Belmont, CA: Brooks/Cole.

Haney, J. H., & Leibsohn, J. (2001). *Basic counseling responses in groups: A multimedia learning system for the helping professions*. Belmont, CA: Brooks/Cole.

Irion, T. (2002). Einsatz von Digitaltechnologien bei der Erhebung, Aufbereitung und Analyse multicodaler Daten. *Forum Qualitative Sozialforschung, 3*(2).

Jacobs, E. E., Masson, R. L., & Harvill, R. L. (1998). *Group counseling: Strategies and skills* (3rd ed.). Pacific Grove, CA: Brooks/Cole.

Koch, S. C., & Zumbach, J. (2002). The use of video analysis software in behavior observation research: Interaction patterns in task-oriented small groups. *Forum Qualitative Sozialforschung, 3*(2).

Kurland, R., & Salmon, R. (1998). *Teaching a methods course in social work with groups*. Alexandria, VA: Council on Social Work Education.

Maple, F. F. (1994). The development of goal-focused interactive videodiscs to enhance student learning in interpersonal practice methods classes. *Computers in Human Services, 11*(3/4), 333-346.

Maypole, D. E. (1991). Interactive videodiscs in social work education. *Social Work, 36*(3), 239-241.

Poulin, J. E., & Walter, C. A. (1990). Interviewing skills and computer assisted instruction: BSW student perceptions. *Computers in Human Services, 7*(3/4), 179-197.

Seabury, B. A., & Maple, F. F. (1993). Using computers to teach practice skills. *Social Work, 38*(4), 430-439.

Shapiro, J. L., Peltz, L. S., & Bernadett-Shapiro, S. (1998). *Brief group treatment: Practical training for therapists and counselors*. Pacific Grove, CA: Brooks/Cole.

Strauss, A. L. (1987). *Qualitative analysis for social scientists*. Cambridge: Cambridge University Press.

Wayne, J. L., & Cohen, C. S. (2001). *Group work education in the field*. Alexandria, VA: Council on Social Work Education.

Weitzman, E. A. (1999). Analyzing qualitative data with computer software. *Health Services Research, 34*(5).

Wodarski, J. S., Bricout, J. C., & Smokowski, P. R. (1996). Making interactive videodisc computer simulation accessible and practice relevant. *Journal of Teaching in Social Work, 13*(1/2), 15-26.

Yalom, I. D. (1975). *The theory and practice of group psychotherapy* (2nd ed.). New York: Basic Books.

Yalom, I. D. (1995). *The theory and practice of group psychotherapy* (4th ed.). New York: Basic Books.

Electronic Advocacy
and Social Welfare Policy Education

Sung Seek Moon

Kevin L. DeWeaver

SUMMARY. The rapid increase in the number of low-cost computers, the proliferation of user-friendly software, and the development of electronic networks have created the "informatics era." The Internet is a rapidly growing communication resource that is becoming mainstream in the American society. Computer-based electronic political advocacy by social workers attempting to influence public policy has proliferated in recent years. Advocacy using high-tech lobbying tools has spread to all social policy debates. Despite this exploration of electronic advocacy, scholars have made little effort to study this area. This paper will discuss the following four dimensions: (1) definition of computer-based electronic advocacy, (2) advantages of computer-based electronic advocacy, (3) challenges of computer-based electronic advocacy, and (4) incorp-

---

Sung Seek Moon, PhD, is Assistant Professor, University of Texas at Arlington. Kevin L. DeWeaver, PhD, is affiliated with the School of Social Work, University of Georgia.

Address correspondence to: Sung Seek Moon, PhD, University of Texas at Arlington, 211 South Cooper Street, BLDG A-208B, Arlington, TX 76019.

[Haworth co-indexing entry note]: "Electronic Advocacy and Social Welfare Policy Education." Moon, Sung Seek, and Kevin L. DeWeaver. Co-published simultaneously in *Journal of Teaching in Social Work* (The Haworth Social Work Practice Press, an imprint of The Haworth Press, Inc.) Vol. 25, No. 1/2, 2005, pp. 57-68; and: *Technology in Social Work Education and Curriculum: The High Tech, High Touch Social Work Educator* (ed: Richard L. Beaulaurier, and Martha Haffey) The Haworth Social Work Practice Press, an imprint of The Haworth Press, Inc., 2005, pp. 57-68. Single or multiple copies of this article are available for a fee from The Haworth Document Delivery Service [1-800-HAWORTH, 9:00 a.m. - 5:00 p.m. (EST). E-mail address: docdelivery@haworthpress.com].

Digital Object Identifier: 10.1300/J067v25n01_04

orating computer-based electronic advocacy into social welfare policy education. *[Article copies available for a fee from The Haworth Document Delivery Service: 1-800-HAWORTH. E-mail address: <docdelivery@haworthpress.com> Website: <http://www.HaworthPress.com>* © *2005 by The Haworth Press, Inc. All rights reserved.]*

KEYWORDS. Advocacy, electronic advocacy, social welfare education, computer, Internet

INTRODUCTION

There is an increasing interest in the use of the Internet and e-mail in the policy-making environment. Interest is increasing, as Klein (1995) has noted; it "facilitates discussion and collective action by citizens, strengthens democracy" (p. 2). Others, such as Richard Davis (1999), have asserted that "Internet is a vehicle for educating individuals, stimulating citizen participation, measuring public opinion, easing citizen access to government officials, offering a public forum, simplifying voter registration, and even facilitating actual voting" (p. 20). *Grohol (1999) reported that an estimated 3.4 trillion e-mail messages were delivered in the U.S.A. in 1998 and that 2.1 billion e-mail messages are sent daily by U.S.A. users.* Denning (1997) argued that the new web-based information technology erodes the four traditional cornerstones of the university: (1) the library as a physical place is soon to be replaced by digital libraries accessible worldwide by almost anyone; (2) the "community of scholars" around the library is soon to be replaced by communities of specialists linked electronically, divorced from geographical location; (3) the ideal-typical small undergraduate class has become unaffordable and is incapable of competing with commercially-provided education on the bases of economics, production values, and entertainment quotient; and (4) job structure has changed such that universities can no longer hope to prepare students for or promise them a "lifelong career," the central selling point until recently. What roles can universities fulfill that people would find valuable? Denning (1997) also addressed that "universities' salvation lay in their ability to use the Internet and information technology as delivery tools while looking for new, primarily adult learners" (p. 29).

Advocacy has been associated with the profession of social work for over 100 years (Gibelman, 1999). Advocacy has been practiced in direct service, case management, administrative, and judicial settings.

Recently, advocacy has been used within the arena of advanced technology. Social work advocacy groups are already using the Internet and e-mail to send targeted messages with information and calls for action around social welfare policy and other issues to those who have electronic mail accounts. The National Association of Social Workers (NASW), for example, uses its discussion list to send out policy announcements and alerts (Fitzgerald & McNutt, 1999). Electronic political advocacy by social workers attempting to influence public policy has proliferated in recent years. Advocacy using high-tech lobbying tools is spreading to all social welfare policy debates. Despite the vast potential of electronic advocacy, scholars have made little effort to study this area. Interestingly, a search of the Social Work Abstracts from 1977-2003 revealed only two articles. Also a review of 12 exemplary human diversity course syllabi published by the Council on Social Work Education (Devore & Fletcher, 1997) revealed that only one contained an Internet application. This paper will describe how the integration of electronic technology can be implemented for social welfare policy after defining electronic advocacy and discussing its advantages as well as its disadvantages.

COMPUTER-BASED ELECTRONIC ADVOCACY

Fitzgerald and McNutt (1999) defined electronic advocacy as "the use of technologically intensive media to influence stakeholders to effect policy change" (p. 334). Increasing numbers of Americans are logging onto the Internet, going "online." An estimated 50 million people used e-mail in 1997, up from an estimated 37 million in 1996 (Davis, 1999). As public notice and use has increased, the Internet increasingly has been accorded an eminent status as the technology of revolutionary change. The Internet and its accompanying e-mail, often called new media advocacy or on-line advocacy, are major tools for approaching policymakers and stakeholders in electronic advocacy (Menon, 2000). Direct mail, telephone campaigns, targeted advertisements, and other forms of mass media are important tools for influencing social welfare policy. However, West and Francis (1996) have questioned the ineffectiveness and limitations of past advocacy specifically related to cost-benefit analysis. For example, television advertising is one of the most powerful tools for advocacy, but it is too expensive for most non-profit social service organizations, as these organizations have limited financial resources. Another limitation of television advertising is its focus on the general public, as opposed to an exclusive focus on decision-makers. How can we overcome these limitations and ineffectiveness? What are alternative approaches? Rees (1998) noted that electronic advocacy can affordably eliminate access barriers and can quickly reach large numbers of people without an enormous financial burden.

ADVANTAGES OF COMPUTER-BASED ELECTRONIC ADVOCACY

Effective policies can be established based on not one-way interaction but two-way communications among policymakers and between policymakers and beneficiaries or stakeholders. Electronic mail (e-mail), which is a main tool for electronic advocacy, has several benefits. Johnson and Huff (2000) noted,

> E-mail uses computer text-processing and communication tools to provide a high-speed information exchange service. The e-mail software on a computer system enables one computer user to communicate with another user or group of users by moving text from one computer mailbox to another. E-mail does not require users to be logged on to the computer at the same time; communication is asynchronous, or non-simultaneous. (p. 520)

The expectation of positive effects of the Internet is to enhance political participation by increasing the quantity of available information for mass participation, and thereby stimulating mobilization (Newhagen & Rafaeli, 1996). *Since their inception, social work organizations have actively sought to bring about social and legal changes concerning the plight of their clients (Mann, 1995; McNutt & Boland, 1998). Web sites on various social and community issues, which social work organizations are concerned about, can provide an inexpensive method to inform the public about laws, policies, and issues of import to a particular agency or community, to publicize national awareness campaigns, and to promote advocacy for social change.* Therefore, many social service agencies and lawmakers involved in policy-making have web sites anyone can access to ask questions, sign petitions, register opinions, or write letters (Tovey, Savicki, & White, 1990). There is evidence that electronic mobilization does facilitate grassroots activity. During the 105th Congress's debate over Internet censorship, one U.S.A. senator's office reported that they received more e-mail messages than phone calls or faxes (Davis, 1999). The Internet and its e-mail are interactive communication technologies. They allow users to receive news and information, as well as to participate in information transmission and public discussion. For example, a bulletin board system on the web site gives a space where individuals can read a proposal, respond, read again, and respond again, while reading input from other participants (Tovey, Savicki, & White, 1990). *Schneider and Lester (2001) noted,*

> *The Internet offers wonderful opportunities that will impact positive social change. Specifically, grassroots organizations and coalitions can network and exchange information in order to (1) obtain funding information and opportunities, (2) obtain information and relevant research, (3) problem-solve with others, and (4) learn about firsthand experiences relating to important issues and problems. (p. 328)*

The Internet also has the advantage of lowering the costs of monitoring politics, organizing group members and other interested individuals, and reaching more persons who are like-minded, but anonymous to the organization (Davis, 1999; Menon, 2000). It potentially diffuses power over information dissemination and public debate. In addition, it extends to overt lobbying by individuals on behalf of their own political interests (Davis, 1999).

Finally, while some may argue against the impersonal nature of computer mediated communication, it has opened doors for persons with disabilities. Johnson and Ashton-Shaeffer (2003) assert that "as computer-mediated communication becomes more commonplace, persons with disabilities will potentially have the opportunity to decrease social isolation and depression, and connect with a cyber community for leisure and social bonding" (p. 77).

CHALLENGES OF COMPUTER-BASED ELECTRONIC ADVOCACY

Social workers and educators should also be alert to the problems and limitations that can be encountered in using technology in advocacy. Although many writers praise the virtues of computer-based advocacy, it is important to note that this electronic frontier also may be dangerous. Some potential challenges are related to the following issues: reliability, accessibility, and privacy/confidentiality.

Reliability. Miller-Cribbs and Chadiha (1998) pointed out that information on the Internet could be inaccurate because a mechanism that would evaluate accuracy in Internet sources does not exist. This means that users need to commit their time to cross-validate Internet information with other written sources to be sure of the facts. *Cornell University Library (2003) offers five criteria for evaluating web resources for credibility as follows*:

1. *Accuracy: Is the information reliable and error-free? Is there an editor or someone who verifies/checks the information?*
2. *Authority: Is there an author? Is the page signed? Is the author qualified? An expert? Who is the sponsor? Is the sponsor of the page reputable? How reputable? Is there a link to information about the author or the sponsor? If the page includes neither a signature nor indicates a sponsor, is there any other way to determine its origin?*
3. *Objectivity: Does the information show a minimum of bias? Is the page designed to sway opinion? Is there any advertising on the page?*
4. *Currency: Is the page dated? If so, when was the last update? How current are the links? Have some expired or moved?*
5. *Coverage: What topics are covered? What does this page offer that is not found elsewhere? What is its intrinsic value? How in-depth is the material?*

Accessibility. Some Internet sites are free and others require a membership fee to access them. Persons with limited resources, and especially those without computers, who may in fact be in more need of services, could be blocked from using these modern resources. According to the Department of Commerce, the Internet useage is highly dependent on income, race, and ethnicity (U. S. Department of Commerce, 1999). Poor and low-income people who cannot afford to buy a computer are limited from using Internet-based social policy advocacy. This implies that many who would be affected by social policy do not have easy access to electronic mail or a Web page (Fitzgerald & McNutt, 1999). Ironically, poor and low-income people are target groups for social welfare policy. Therefore, we need their participation and feedback more than any other groups. The use of community networks is one way for marginalized populations to access electronic systems for reviewing social welfare policies. Non-profit organizations can also receive network access via a community network.

Privacy/Confidentiality. As in electronic service process, confidentiality is a central ethical concern (Sampson, Kolodinsky, & Greeno, 1997; Butterfield, 1995). The social worker has no way of knowing who is in the room with the client when either sending or receiving e-mail. Clients could be at risk without the social worker's knowledge. For example, if an abused woman's batterer has access to her e-mail and can read the interactions of counseling, what is the potential for harm to her? A social worker could violate confidentiality by using transcriptions of sessions in a research report or conference presentation and fail to get consent of the client because of ease of printing out the sessions (Banach & Bernat, 2000; Giffords, 1998). This is a challenging area where extra caution has to be taken to preserve confidentiality and thus protect social workers' clients.

Legitimacy of e-mail. There is some evidence that a lot of policymakers ritualistically ignore e-mails related to advocacy of various social work persons or agencies. How can we make our e-mails look legitimate, not as spam? At least partially, what is and isn't spam is in the eye of the beholder. This implies that advocates should consider some tips:

1. *Subject header of the e-mail should be appropriate and professional: one of the antispam solutions which currently has been developed is to block mails based on keywords in subject line. It is wise to avoid any word alluding to an advertisement or commercial solicitations.*
2. *Do not send a standard message to a large list of policymakers; instead make personalized mail and send it to one person without a large list of names.*
3. *Use agency e-mail address: it can be a possible way of attracting policymakers to check mails based on the professional organization. Its suffix (.edu, .org, .gov, .com) tells them about agency orientation.*
4. *Use "high priority" signal: Sean Lanham, information technology security manager of the University of Texas at Arlington, reported, based on his observations that few spam used a "high priority" signal. He also said that he usually checks mails with a "high priority" signal (personal communication, July 11, 2003).*

INCORPORATING COMPUTER-BASED
ELECTRONIC ADVOCACY
INTO SOCIAL WELFARE POLICY EDUCATION

Social workers work for the best interest of vulnerable populations. This is best accomplished by integrating advanced technologies into traditional advocacy tools. The major challenges facing social work education systems, especially related to social policy in the "informatics era," include issues of how to prepare for and capitalize on the advanced technology and how to integrate computer technology into social work practice. Social welfare policy is sensitive to the current social, political, environmental, economic, or technological changes. Without the sense of recognizing and using those changes, professionals cannot perform their job effectively. Social workers do not need to be experts in all areas, but do need to possess minimal competencies in advanced technology.

The Internet and e-mail should not replace traditional forms of advocacy. Certainly, electronic advocacy alone cannot help our clients. However, computer-based electronic advocacy can be used to contact a wider range of available sources including individuals, agencies, and newsgroups to impact social welfare policy-making. It is an important mission to incorporate these techniques in both policy practice and the teaching of social welfare policy. How can we incorporate these new technologies into social welfare policy education? Cnaan (1989) suggested the following ways:

1. Educate students in information technology applications, and not in programming;
2. Provide broad-based knowledge that graduates can build on to meet the requirements of their employers;
3. Update curricula periodically so that students' educating can be kept current;
4. Match information technology curricula with the agencies' needs based on empirical data; and
5. Incorporate information technology into core courses rather than into a separate technical course (pp. 237-238).

Schools of social work should provide students with the necessary computer skills including how to develop a web site that features original research and links to resources, and how to manage a web site. This type of effort is easy to create and serves as a resource for many stakeholders. Students need skills to conduct a survey or disseminate necessary information by using the Internet or e-mail. Fitzgerald and McNutt (1999) asserted that "information literacy skills can be taught in cooperation with social work librarians" (p. 337). They further stated,

> Information literacy provides a means to separate credible materials from those that are less helpful. Students need skills in using a Web browser, employing search engines, critiquing courses, and using critical thinking skills to evaluate information. (p. 337)

Next, schools of social work should develop workshops or training programs based on the needs assessment for faculty members who are not familiar with advanced technologies (Peart & Sheffield, 2001). Marson (1997) asserted that workshops and training programs must be freely offered in a non-intimidating manner. The workshops or training programs can help the faculty to have a deeper understanding and ability to evaluate and use them. Sliwa (1994) suggested that instructors should resist the temptation to embrace all available technology without question. Johnson and Huff (2000) asserted that educators are encouraged to accept only those strategies that improve the quality of learning and to evaluate carefully any technological tools they choose to use in the classroom. The workshop and training program may be a great opportunity for examining several technological tools for implementing social welfare policy education.

Schools of social work also need to establish a guideline to protect students and social agencies from negative consequences inherent in a highly computerized society. Cnaan (1989) pointed out three major threats to society: (1) widening the gap between the stronger and the weaker in society; (2) curtailing individual freedom consequent on enhanced mechanisms of social control; and (3) disrupting traditional social standards and relationships and replacing them with new rules or creating anomie (p. 239). A guideline should be established by an in-depth study that could include the societal impacts of information technology and the traditional role of social work and information technology.

In addition, schools of social work should provide students several opportunities to practice some types of electronic advocacy. For instance, the University of Georgia School of Social Work requires students to attend a NASW Lobby Day and then e-mail their local congressman about an issue or, preferably, a bill that may become a law or one they do not want to become a law. Roberts Wesleyan College Division of Social Work also requires a community and organization class where students find a germane advocacy web site (e.g., moveon. org) and post a relevant social issue on the board or respond to any of the ongoing campaigns and report their involvement and progress once a week as one of class assignments.

Finally, it is necessary to establish appropriate ethical standards for Internet on-line social work services. Even though the National Association of Social Workers (NASW) has the Code of Ethics addressing general ethical guidelines for social workers, electronic-based social work services require more specific and applicable rules to follow in conjunction with the Code of Ethics. Ethical standards for Internet on-line services should address several aspects, such as privacy information, informational notices, client waiver, records of electronic communications, electronic transfer of client information, appropriateness of on-line service, service plan, continuing coverage, boundaries of competence, minor or incompetent clients, and legal considerations (Bloom & Walz, 2000).

CONCLUSION

This paper has discussed electronic advocacy and its implication for social welfare policy education, along with describing the advantages and challenges of electronic advocacy. It is imperative that social workers begin to use the advanced technologies for effective social policy advocacy. As practitioners use these technologies, they must carefully consider the implication issues, especially their impact on individual clients, agencies, and stakeholders. Also, regarding social work practitioners, it should not be assumed that they know how to use the technology discussed here; indeed, this is an empirical research question that needs some study. What such a study would probably show is a vast diversity in social workers' computer skills. The question then becomes how practitioners can be taught basic computer skills for electronic advocacy. One possible answer is that the Schools of Social Work could offer various continuing education options, which could last from one evening to several weeks or even occur on weekends.

Further study is recommended to determine the number of social work programs that teach electronic advocacy in both BSW and MSW programs and investigate the desire of students and social work organizations to use these tools. We also need to determine the implementation issues (e.g., lack of financial resources and expertise) confronting those social work education programs which have expanded to social welfare policy education with advanced technologies. Finally, it is recommended that a model program to use electronic advocacy be developed, implemented, and evaluated; the results of this effort would go a long way to speak to the interest that has been created heretofore.

REFERENCES

Abramson, J. B., Arterton, F. C., & Orren, G. R. (1988). *The electronic commonwealth: The impact of new media technologies on democratic politics.* New York: Basic Books.

Banach, M., & Bernat, F. P. (2000). Liability and the Internet: Risks and recommendations for social work practice. *Journal of Technology in Human Services, 17,* 153-171.

Bloom, J. W., & Walz, G. R. (Eds.) (2000). *Cybercounseling and cyberlearning: Strategies and resources for the millennium.* Alexander, VA: American Counseling Association.

Butterfield, W. H. (1995). Computer utilization. In R. L. Edwards (Ed.-in-Chief), *Encyclopedia of social work* (19th ed., pp. 594-613). Washington, DC: NASW Press.

Cnaan, R. A. (1989). Social work education and direct practice in the computer age. *Journal of Social Work Education, 25,* 235-243.

Cornell University Library (2003). Evaluating web sites: Criteria and tools [On-line]. Available Internet: *http://www.library.cornell.edu/okuref/research/webeval.html*

Davis, R. (1999). *The web of politics: The Internet's impact on the American political system.* New York: Oxford University Press.

Denning, P. J. (1996). The university's next challenges. *Communications of the ACM, 39* (5), 27-31.

Devore, W., & Fletcher, B. (1997). *Human diversity content in social work education.* Alexandria, VA: Council on Social Work Education.

Fitzgerald, E., & McNutt, J. (1999). Electronic advocacy in policy practice: A framework for teaching technologically based practice. *Journal of Social Work Education, 35,* 331-341.

Gibelman, M. (1999). The search for identity: Defining social work–Past, present, future. *Social Work, 44,* 298-310.

Giffords, E. D. (1998). Social work on the internet: An introduction. *Social Work, 43,* 243-251.

Grohol, J. (1999). Best practices in e-therapy: Confidentiality & privacy [On-line]. Available Internet: *http://www.ismho.org/issues/19901.htm*

Johnson, D., & Ashton-Shaeffer, C. (2003, March). Virtual buddies: Using computer-mediated communication in therapeutic recreation. *Parks & Recreation,* 77-79.

Johnson, M., & Huff, M. T. (2000). Students' use of computer-mediated communication in a distance education course. *Research on Social Work Practice, 10,* 519-532.

Klein, H. K. (1995). *Grassroots democracy and the Internet: The telecommunications policy roundtable-Northeast (TPR-NE)* [On-line]. Available: *http://ralph.gmu.edu/~pbaker/klein.txt*

Latting, J. K. (1994). Diffusion of computer-mediated communication in a graduate social work class: Lessons from "The class from hell." *Computers in Human Services, 10* (3), 21-45.

Laurillard, D. (1993). *Rethinking university teaching: A framework for the effective use of educational technology.* London: Routledge.

Margetts, H. (1999). *Information technology in government.* New York: Routledge.

Marson, S. M. (1997). A selective history of Internet technology and social work. *Computers and Human Services, 14,* 35-49.

Menon, G. M. (2000). The 79-cent campaign: The use of on-line mailing lists for electronic advocacy. *Journal of Community Practice, 8,* 73-81.

Miller-Cribbs, J. E., & Chadiha, L. A. (1998). Integrating the internet in a human diversity course. *Computers in Human Services. 15,* 97-108.

Newhagen, J., & Sheizaf, R. (1996, Winter). Why communication researchers should study the Internet. *Journal of Communication, 46,* 1-12.

Peart, M., & Sheffield, C. J. (2001). Technology training for teacher education in Jamaica: A case for needs assessment. *Computers in the Schools, 18,* 151-164.

Rash, W. (1997). *Politics on the nets: Writing the political process.* New York: W. H. Freeman.

Rees, S. (1998). *Effective non-profit advocacy.* Washington, DC: Aspen Institute.

Sampson, J. P., Jr., Kolodinsky, R. W., & Greeno, B. P. (1997). Counseling on the information highway: Future possibilities and potential problems. *Journal of Counseling and Development, 75,* 203-212.

Schneider, R. L., & Lester, L. (2001). *A new framework for action: Social work advocacy.* Belmont, CA: Brooks/Cole.

Sliwa, S. (1994). Re-engineering the learning process with information technology. *Academe, 80,* 8-12.

Tovey, R., Savicki, V., & White, C. (1990). Electronic networking in human service agencies: A developmental analysis. *Child Welfare, 69,* 115-128.

U. S. Department of Commerce (1999). *Falling through the net: Defining the digital divide.* Washington, DC: Author.

West, D. M., & Francis, R. (1996). Electronic advocacy: Internet groups and public policy-making. *PS: Political Science and Politics, 29* (2), 25-29.

Assessing the Virtual Classroom of a Graduate Social Policy Course

Maria Roberts-DeGennaro
John Clapp

SUMMARY. Student perceptions were investigated toward their experience of learning online in a web-based graduate social policy course. Overall, student perceptions were positive toward the online features of this course with the most useful features being the PowerPoint lecture notes and the Discussion Board. Students were more satisfied with their interactions with the instructor than with the other students. A majority of the students reported they would take another online course and would also recommend this specific course to other students. Female students were more likely to ask for technical assistance. Students enjoyed learning as much through the virtual classroom as a traditional on-campus section of the course. *[Article copies available for a fee from The Haworth Document Delivery Service: 1-800-HAWORTH. E-mail address: <docdelivery@haworthpress.com> Website: <http://www.HaworthPress.com> © 2005 by The Haworth Press, Inc. All rights reserved.]*

Maria Roberts-DeGennaro, PhD, Professor, and John Clapp, PhD, Professor, are affiliated with the School of Social Work, San Diego State University, San Diego, CA 92182.

Address correspondence to: Maria Roberts-DeGennaro, PhD, School of Social Work, San Diego State University, 5500 Campanile Drive, San Diego, CA 92182 (E-mail: mdegenna@mail.sdsu.edu).

[Haworth co-indexing entry note]: "Assessing the Virtual Classroom of a Graduate Social Policy Course." Roberts-DeGennaro, Maria, and John Clapp. Co-published simultaneously in *Journal of Teaching in Social Work* (The Haworth Social Work Practice Press, an imprint of The Haworth Press, Inc.) Vol. 25, No. 1/2, 2005, pp. 69-88; and: *Technology in Social Work Education and Curriculum: The High Tech, High Touch Social Work Educator* (ed: Richard L. Beaulaurier, and Martha Haffey) The Haworth Social Work Practice Press, an imprint of The Haworth Press, Inc., 2005, pp. 69-88. Single or multiple copies of this article are available for a fee from The Haworth Document Delivery Service [1-800-HAWORTH, 9:00 a.m. - 5:00 p.m. (EST). E-mail address: docdelivery@haworthpress.com].

Digital Object Identifier: 10.1300/J067v25n01_05

KEYWORDS. Social policy, distance education, virtual classroom, computers, technology, web-based course, online learning, computer-mediated instruction

RATIONALE

The technology revolution in higher education is challenging social work educators to create new pedagogical strategies, particularly in response to the growing demand for electronic pedagogy. Sonwalkar (2001) contends that the instructional design for constructing a web-based course is still an art form, primarily because of the variations in the nature of course content both within and across disciplines. Models that are appropriate for course material are numerous, and there exists a wide range of possibilities for structuring a course.

In response to the developments in integrating telecommunications and computer technologies, educational theory is shifting to a constructivist conception of learning. Based on this framework, learners are responsible for constructing meaning, as well as engaging in authentic reciprocal communication for the purposes of confirming understanding and generating worthwhile knowledge (Anderson & Garrison, 1998). Thus, the challenge for distance educators is to set up a cognitively rich learning environment to facilitate the learner's constructive processes (Zhang, 1998).

Raymond and Pike (1997, p. 282) suggest that the use of technologies for teaching purposes will require a paradigm shift. We will need to rethink the nature of higher education, roles of teachers and students, physical environment in which learning occurs, and issues related to intellectual property. Students will be expected to take on a more proactive role, assuming increasing responsibility for their own learning. The instructor will serve as a facilitator or enabler rather than a purveyor of information.

Traditionally, relationships in higher education were viewed as interactions between teacher, student, and content. Moore (1989) suggested three interactions emerged from these relationships: (a) learner-teacher, (b) learner-content, and (c) learner-learner. In contrast, Garrison (1989) suggested the educational transaction could be viewed as overlapping triadic relationships with six possible types of interactions. In this latter model, at the intersection of three macro-components, three interactions exist: (a) learner-teacher, (b) learner-content, and (c) teacher-content.

Then, within these three macro-components, another set of interactions exist: (a) learner-learner, (b) teacher-teacher, and (c) content-content.

With the rapid increase in the growth of distance education, particularly in computer-mediated instructional methods, a reconceptualization of traditional teaching-learning transactions is emerging that recognizes the interactive capabilities of communication technologies. Anderson and Garrison (1998, p. 110) contend that learning in a networked world presents many new roles and responsibilities for both the teacher and the learner. It will radically change the construction and delivery of the course content in higher education.

In turn, this will stimulate research to examine the quality of the relationships between instructors and students when using new types of instructional methodologies, such as electronic pedagogical models (Harrington, 1999). In addition, there will be a demand for assessing learning outcomes from technology-driven distance education that allows courses to become increasingly learner-centered (Hodes, 1997-98). Palloff and Pratt (1999) believe that evaluating outcomes, both in terms of the learning process and learner satisfaction with the course, is a more complex process in the virtual classroom.

Raymond, Ginsberg and Gohagan (1998) suggest that the use of web-based technology in providing a venue for teaching outside of the traditional on-campus classroom is pushing the boundaries of distance education definitions. Thus, a challenge in distance education is to develop appropriate learning experiences so that the methods and technology match the learner's needs. Hantula (1998) suggests that the technology should not necessarily limit or facilitate teaching a particular subject. Rather, the technology must be assembled and managed to meet the expected learning outcomes of the course. For example, Sieppert and Krysik (1996) contend that computer-based testing is a viable and worthwhile endeavor for social work educators to explore in assessing learning outcomes and in developing curriculum content.

Siegel, Jennings, Conklin and Flynn's (1998) national survey of accredited social work programs revealed that the most frequently delivered distance education courses in MSW programs were policy courses and electives. In contrast, BSW programs primarily offered research, human behavior and the social environment, and methods courses through distance learning. Both sets of programs reported the use of distance learning in conducting seminars for field educators.

Crook and Brady (1998) found little empirical evidence about the effectiveness of either computer-assisted instruction or web-based instruction in social work education. Stocks and Freddolino (1998) compared a web-based graduate research methods course with an on-campus section of the course. They found that student performance was comparable in both sections. Likewise, Royse (2000) taught a web-based research methods course in a MSW program and compared it to traditional on-campus sections of the course. He concluded that students learned about as much research content in the web-based class as students in a traditional on-campus classroom.

Harrington (1999) compared a graduate level statistics course that was taught using software-based content with an on-campus section of the course. Findings from the latter study suggested that students who previously were academically successful could do as well in statistics with a programmed instructional approach as students in a traditional classroom course.

Seaberg (1999) taught two sequential clinical research courses as virtual classroom courses for MSW students in a clinical concentration. Based on this virtual classroom experience, he believes that course materials can be prepared and presented on an Internet website for online learning. It is crucial, however, that these materials are easy for students to use and sufficiently clear and complete.

Stocks and Freddolino (2000) evaluated two iterations of an Internet-based graduate social work research course. Their study concluded that the more opportunities for interactivity are built into the course, the easier it is to create an active learning environment for the students.

In the evolution of developing paradigms for electronic pedagogy, an informed debate is needed to continue about effective virtual (any-place-anytime) technologies and the practice of using these technologies (Graves, 2000). An important step in furthering the development of using technology and in formulating online teaching models is to increase the experiential base of a variety of faculty testing the virtual classroom on a variety of content areas with a variety of students (Seaberg, 1999).

Palloff and Pratt (1999) contend that it is important to receive feedback from students in a virtual classroom on their overall experience of working online through the institution. Different forms of evaluation might occur such as: (a) evaluation of student performance, (b) evaluation of the course and the quality of instruction, and (c) evaluation of the technology being used, including its functionality and user friendliness. All of these forms of evaluation should lead to an ongoing process of planning and review so that online courses can be continuously improved. Therefore, faculty must be expected to provide feedback on their experience of teaching in the online environment, in order to contribute to the knowledge base of using electronic pedagogy.

The purpose of this present study is to investigate student perceptions toward their experience of learning online in a web-based graduate social policy course in the School of Social Work at San Diego State University. This investigation considered multiple sources of data in evaluating how students experienced online learning in two web-based sections of this course. The study also compared the learning outcomes based on average course grades and course evaluation ratings between the two web-based sections and one section of the course that was taught in a traditional on-campus classroom.

Social policy is a foundation course that first-year graduate students are required to complete during the first semester of their graduate program in the School. The first author taught two web-based sections of this course during the Fall 2001 semester through the Blackboard Software Platform: (a) one section of 23 students registered for the course on the main campus, which is located in an urban, metropolitan community; and (b) one section of 23 students registered for the course on the branch campus, located in a rural and predominantly Hispanic community. The traditional on-campus section of the course consisted of 22 students who registered for the course on the main campus.

OVERVIEW OF WEB-BASED COURSE

The web-based graduate social policy course was constructed and pilot-tested by the first author in Fall 2000. Graduated implementation of a web-based course is an effective way for educators to gain experience in online teaching and to evaluate the suitability of the course for online learning (Knowles, 2001). In a previous article, Roberts-DeGennaro (2002) describes the framework of a constructivist conception of learning that was used in designing this web-based course. A topic-driven syllabus was developed for the course, in which there was a weekly schedule that included a range of topics with required readings geared to those topics. In both web-based sections, the course objectives, content, and assignments were the same.

Based on the weekly schedule, a PowerPoint presentation of lecture materials with graphics was created by the instructor for each week. At the beginning of each presentation, the weekly required readings were posted along with reminders of assignments that were due in the near future. Then, a set of PowerPoint lecture notes was presented that addressed the weekly topics, as well as active links to World Wide Web sites providing additional information related to the course materials. On the last slide, a few study questions appeared which raised issues that were addressed in the lecture notes or required readings. These weekly PowerPoint presentations remained available on the web-based course so that students could refer back to these over the semester.

The instructor produced six video clips so that every other week during the semester an electronic audio-visual communication was available to the students. The purpose of these video clips was to provide a personal message from the instructor. The first video clip was an orientation to the course. The other video clips were instructions for completing the course assignments that reinforced written information describing these assignments in the online courseware materials. In addition, written transcripts of these video clips were accessible on the web-based course. Web content accessibility guidelines were used in developing the course content (Sarnoff, 2001; W3C, 1999).

In the virtual classroom, the instructor posted announcements, such as reminders about due dates for assignments, schedule for chat sessions, etc., on a regular basis. One-hour chat sessions were scheduled every other week during the semester as office hours in cyberspace. These chat sessions provided an opportunity for the students, if they wanted to interact with the instructor through synchronous electronic communication.

Three online quizzes were administered about a month apart during the semester. The purpose of these quizzes was not only to assist the students in reviewing the course materials, but also to prepare for the qualifying examination that the students are expected to successfully pass in their graduate program.

As one of the assignments, the students were required to investigate a bill that would either affect existing social policy or propose new social policy legislation. This bill was expected to be under debate either at the state or federal level of government. It was expected to have a direct impact on the provision, planning and/or evaluation of health and human services in the United States. The instructor provided a framework for the students to use in analyzing the proposed legislation, as well as 20 active links to World Wide Web sites to assist the students in researching the proposed legislation. Students were required to cite references consisting of government documents, refereed publications, World Wide Web sites, and other sources in the social policy analysis. Then the students submitted this social policy analysis as an attachment in an e-mail message to the instructor.

After completing this social policy analysis, the students were required to engage in electronic advocacy by preparing a statement to either support or oppose the proposed legislation and submitting it as an e-mail message to their elected representative(s). The instructor provided a set of active links to World Wide Web sites to assist the students in identifying their representatives. In addition, the instructor provided a framework that the students were expected to use in preparing this electronic advocacy assignment. A copy of the e-mail message, when it was sent to the representative, was required to be sent to the instructor as evidence of completing the assignment.

Students were required to add a discussion thread to 10 forums, such as Faith-Based and Community Initiatives, Re-Authorization of Welfare Reform Legislation, etc., on the Discussion Board. Posting discussion threads to a forum on the Discussion Board was important in facilitating interaction among the students. The students were required to either express their viewpoint or raise a question related to a particular forum in their discussion thread. The students were required to document at least 10 forums in which they started a discussion thread and then e-mail this list to the instructor. The instructor confirmed this list by checking the online record of discussion threads to each forum.

Finally, the students were required to create a Homepage on the web-based course. These Homepages provided an avenue for the students to share some personal information, as well as an opportunity for the students to use computer technology in uploading an appropriate photograph or a piece of graphic art. In addition, students were expected to post information on the Homepage related to the proposed piece of legislation that they were analyzing.

METHODOLOGY

Subjects

Recruitment Methods

An announcement regarding the option to enroll in the web-based course section was disseminated to new students who were accepted by the University into the graduate social work program. The instructor, who taught the web-based class sections, recruited student participation from students who had registered for the web-based section on the main campus (urban), and from students who had registered for the web-based section on the branch campus (rural), at an orientation to the course during the first week of classes in the Fall 2001 semester. Students in the traditional on-campus course section did have an option to register for the web-based section, but chose to register for the traditional on-campus course section. The fact that the student subjects were not randomly assigned to the course sections is a limitation of the study.

RESEARCH DESIGN

Research Questions

This descriptive, evaluative study was designed to examine the following research questions:

- What are the perceptions of students toward the online features of a web-based course?
- What are the attitudes of students in a web-based course toward the learner-content, learner-learner, and learner-instructor interactions?
- Did the learning outcomes based on average course grade and course evaluation ratings differ among students in a web-based course and a traditional on-campus section of the course?

Instruments

The Assessment of Computer-Mediated Instruction Form

The Assessment of Computer-Mediated Instruction Form was constructed and pilot-tested by the first author to describe the attitudes of the students who completed the web-based course toward the teaching-learning transactions, and their perceptions toward the online features of the course. This instrument measured the following domains: (a) attitudes toward the usefulness of the online course features, (b) attitudes toward the usefulness of the course assignments, and (c) attitudes concerning student satisfaction with learner-learner and learner-instructor interactions. The form contains several Likert-type items with open-ended follow-up questions. The open-ended items were analyzed qualitatively by the researchers and coded numerically.

Demographic Background Information Form

A Demographic Background Information Form was constructed and then pilot tested by the first author for collecting data on personal and demographic information. The following variables were used to describe the characteristics between students in the rural and the urban class sections: age, gender, racial/ethnic background, Bachelor's Degree major, use of computer at previous paid employment experiences, use of computer in previous courses, access to computer with modem at home, had an e-mail account during previous year, current semester unit load, enrolled in a field practicum during current semester, hours a week working in a paid position during current semester, number of years of paid social work practice experience, time spent traveling between place of residence and campus, number of years using a computer, hours a week using a computer, and completion of an online college course.

Learning Outcomes

The final course grades for each of the three course sections were used in assessing the learning achieved by the students at the end of the semester. In addition, a standard Course Evaluation Instrument that was developed through the University was administered at the end of the semester to assess the students' experience of the course and the material they studied. This Instrument collected data for calculating the following ratings: (a) average rating for the course overall, (b) average rating for the teacher's contribution to the course, and (c) average rating for the effectiveness of the course.

Procedure

Students in both sections of the web-based course were administered the Demographic Background Information Form at the on-campus orientation to the course during the first week of classes in the Fall 2001 semester. Likewise, the students in the traditional on-campus section were administered the Demographic Background Information Form during their first class session in the Fall 2001 semester. It took the students about 10 minutes to complete this Form.

Students in both sections of the web-based course were administered the Assessment of Computer-Mediated Instruction Form at a second on-campus class session which was held during the last week of the Fall

2001 semester. It took the students about 20 minutes to complete this Form.

An average course grade was calculated for each of the three course sections by the instructor through using the final course grades that were earned by students at the end of the Fall 2001 semester. Students could earn a grade of "A," "B," "C," "D," or "F."

The Course Evaluation Instrument was administered to students in both sections of the web-based course at the aforementioned second on-campus class session and to students in the traditional on-campus course during their last class session in the Fall 2001 semester. It took the students about 15 minutes to complete this Instrument.

ANALYSIS AND RESULTS

Sample

There was a more equal gender distribution in the rural branch web-based section than in either the main urban web-based section or the traditional on-campus section: (a) 13 (56.5%) female, 10 (43.5%) male in the rural branch web-based section; (b) 19 (83%) female, 4 (17%) male in the main urban web-based section; and (c) 18 (82%) female, 4 (18%) male in the traditional on-campus section.

The main urban web-based section and the traditional on-campus section were more ethnically diverse than the rural branch web- based section, which consisted of 22 (96%) Hispanic students and one student whose ethnic/racial grouping was reported as "Other." This finding was expected since the students in the rural branch web-based section reside in a predominantly Hispanic community. In contrast, the main urban web-based section represented the following groups: (a) 14 (61%) Caucasian non-Hispanic, (b) 3 (13%) Hispanic, (c) 2 (9%) Black/African-American, (d) 3 (13%) Asian/ Asian Pacific, and (e) 1 (4%) "Other." The traditional on-campus section represented the following groups: (a) 11 (50%) Caucasian non- Hispanic, (b) 8 (36%) Hispanic, (c) 1 (4.55%) Black/African-American, (d) 1 (4.55%) Asian/ Asian Pacific, and (e) 1 (4.55%) "Other."

Across all three sections, the average age was 31.8 years (SD = 8.9). The average age for each of the sections was fairly similar: (a) Mean = 32.0 years, SD = 10.0 for the main urban web-based section; (b) Mean = 32.3 years, SD = 7.3 for the rural branch web-based section; and (c) Mean = 31.0 years, SD = 9.5 for the traditional on-campus section.

Nearly half (n = 33) of the 68 students had majored in the field of psychology for their Bachelor's Degree. Only about 15% (n = 10) of these students had majored in the field of social work. The remaining (n = 25) students had majored in a variety of fields.

On the average, students in the rural branch web-based section were working 40 (SD = 10.0) hours per week in a paid position and taking 6 course units (two courses). In contrast, the students in the main urban web-based section on average were working 20 (SD = 15.5) hours per week and taking 12 course units (four courses); and the students in the traditional on-campus section on average were working 27 (SD = 16.4) hours per week and taking 9 course units (three courses). Depending on the nature of the paid position, it appears that the average weekly work/course load was fairly similar across the three sections.

Findings

Computer Experience

At the beginning of their graduate program of study, the students in the traditional on-campus section reported using a computer for more years than students in the two web-based sections: (a) Mean = 8.2 years, SD = 3.5 for the main urban web-based section; (b) Mean = 7.3 years, SD = 3.6 for the rural branch web-based section; and (c) Mean = 10.3, SD = 4.6 for the traditional on-campus section.

Likewise, at the beginning of their graduate program of study, the students in the traditional on-campus section reported using a computer for more hours per week than students in the two web-based sections: (a) Mean = 12.5 hours, SD = 15.0 for the main urban web-based section; (b) Mean = 17.4 hours, SD = 14.1 for the rural branch web-based section; and (c) Mean = 18.0 hours, SD = 13.4 for the traditional on-campus section.

Student Ratings of Online Features

Table 1 presents the ratings by students toward various online features of the web-based course. Overall, students found the PowerPoint lecture notes (Mean = 3.6, SD = .7) and the Discussion Board (Mean = 3.6, SD = .6) to be the most useful features of the course. Over 70% (n = 33) of the students viewed the video clips that were accessible on the web-based course, and of these latter students, 60.9% found them to be

TABLE 1. Student Ratings of the Utility of Online Course Features (N = 46)

Online Course Feature	Usefulness							
	Great Extent		Some Extent		No Extent		Not Used/ Uncertain	
	n	%	n	%	n	%	n	%
Chat Room	5	10.9	9	19.6	1	2.2	31	67.4
Discussion Board	32	69.6	12	26.1	1	2.2	1	2.2
Video Clips	9	19.6	19	41.3	5	10.9	13	28.3
PowerPoint	31	67.4	13	28.3	0	0	2	4.3

useful. The majority of students (67.4%) did not participate in the chat sessions.

To learn more about the above ratings, students were asked to elaborate on their ratings for each of the online course features in an open-ended question. The open-ended responses were then coded into common categories by the investigators.

The PowerPoint lecture notes were viewed by 95.7% (n = 44) of the students as either being useful to a "great extent" (n = 31) or to "some extent" (n = 13). Students reported the online PowerPoint presentations primarily served two functions. First, the presentations provided a tool for reviewing the course materials and studying for the quizzes (n = 24, 52.2%). Second, the presentations provided a clear source of information related to the course content (n = 21, 45.7%).

Interestingly, 95.7% (n = 44) of the students also viewed the Discussion Board as either being useful to a "great extent" (n = 32) or to "some extent" (n = 12). Most (n = 40) of the students reported that the Discussion Board was useful because it provided opportunities to learn and share information with the other students.

Over sixty percent (n = 28) of the students perceived the video clips to be useful. The qualitative comments regarding the online video clips were mixed. Notably, 15 students (32.6%) reported that the video clips served as an important reminder to students about course assignments and requirements. Ten (21.7%) of the students reported that these clips provided a sense of connectedness to the instructor. Despite these positive comments, 19.6% (n = 9) of the students reported that reading the written transcripts of the videos was an easier way of accessing the same material.

Comments concerning the chat sessions were also mixed. About a third (n = 15) of the students reported that these sessions were scheduled at inconvenient times, even though the instructor polled the students as to their preferred times for scheduling the sessions. Almost another third (n = 14) of the students reported that participation in the chat sessions provided an opportunity to network with other students in the course. About a fourth (n = 11) of the students reported that participation in the chat sessions was too time consuming.

Interactions and Technical Assistance

Although the students enrolled in the course were, for the most part, computer savvy, 47.8% (n = 22) of the students sought out technical assistance during the semester. Table 2 depicts the sources of assistance including: (a) instructor (30.4%); (b) online student manual (15.2%); (c) University's Instructional Technology Services' web site for Blackboard (4.3%); and (d) Other sources (21.7%), which were primarily friends, family members, and co-workers.

Students were also asked to rate their level of satisfaction with the interactions they had with both the instructor and other students in the web-based course. Ninety-eight percent (n = 45) of the students reported to be satisfied either to "some extent" (56.5%) or to a "great extent" (41.3%) with their interactions with the instructor. Yet, in an open-ended question asking students to discuss their frustrations with the course, 10 students (21.7%) reported that they would have liked to have more interaction with the instructor.

In contrast, eighty percent (n = 37) of the students reported to be satisfied either to "some extent" (47.8%) or to a "great extent" (32.6%)

TABLE 2. Student Ratings of Sources for Technical Assistance (N = 46)

Source of Assistance	Sought Technical Assistance			
	Yes		No	
	n	%	n	%
Instructor	14	30.4	32	69.6
Student Manual Online	7	15.2	39	84.8
Instructional Technology Services	2	4.3	44	95.7
Other	10	21.7	36	78.3

with their interactions with other students in the course. Seven students (15.2%) were not satisfied with their level of interaction with the other students in the web-based course section and two (4.3%) students were "uncertain."

All (N = 46) of the students rated the social policy analysis assignment as increasing their knowledge of the legislative process either to "some extent" (19.6%) or to a "great extent" (80.4%). Likewise, 96% (n = 44) of the students rated the electronic advocacy assignment either to "some extent" (21.7%) or to a "great extent" (73.9%) as increasing their understanding of policy advocacy.

Finally, when students were asked whether they would take another online course, over 90% (n = 42) of the students reported they would enroll in another online course. Only four students reported that they were "uncertain" about enrolling in another online course. In an open-ended follow-up question, 63% (n = 29) of the students reported that the flexibility of the online course was an important factor towards contributing to their desire to take another online course.

Along similar lines, students were asked to describe any new learning that they achieved as a result of completing the web-based course. Sixty-one percent (n = 28) reported that they learned about new online data sources. Thirty-seven percent (n = 17) reported that they gained confidence in using computer technology.

In addition to the above univariate analyses, we examined the data for differences by class section (main campus vs. rural branch campus) and gender. We also examined whether past computer experience was related to satisfaction with the course. The only statistically significant difference found was that females were more likely to ask for technical assistance than were their male counterparts (t = 3.0, df = 43.3, p = .005).

Learning Outcomes

Learning outcomes by the three course sections are reported in Table 3. As shown in this Table, none of the course sections varied significantly on any of the learning outcomes. Overall, students in each section performed at a "B" grade-level in the three course sections. A grade of "B" for a graduate course is considered an "average" grade for graduate-level courses in the University.

The means values from the student ratings were all in the "Above Average" range on the standard Course Evaluation Instrument including: (a) average rating for course overall, (b) average rating for the teacher's

TABLE 3. Learning Outcomes by Course Section

Outcome	Web-Based Main Campus N = 23 Mean	Web-Based Rural Branch Campus N = 23 Mean	On-Campus Classroom Main Campus N = 22 Mean
Course Grade*	3.48	3.40	3.32
Student Rating of Course Overall**	4.28	4.23	4.25
Student Rating of Teacher's Contribution**	4.19	4.33	4.30
Student Rating of Course Effectiveness**	4.38	4.14	4.21

Note: The course sections do not statistically differ on any of the learning outcomes.
*Course Grading Scale: 4.0 = A, 3.0 = B, 2.0 = C, 1.0 = D
**Course Evaluation Rating Scale: 5 = Outstanding, 4 = Above Average, 3 = Average, 2 = Below Average, 1 = Poor

contribution to the course, and (c) average rating for the effectiveness of the course. Thus, the two web-based course sections and the traditional on-campus course section were equally well received by the students. An "Above Average" rating would be expected of a graduate-level course in the University.

DISCUSSION

The most useful online features of the web-based course were the PowerPoint lecture notes and the Discussion Board. The students perceived the PowerPoint lecture notes as a tool for reviewing the course materials and studying for quizzes, as well as being a clear source of information related to the course content. This finding is in sharp contrast with Schoech's (2000) study in which only a few of the eight student subjects liked the use of PowerPoint presentations in his web-based practice course. Nevertheless, Seaberg's (2001) survey of the use of the Internet and other teaching tools in graduate social work education revealed that the most commonly used computer-based teaching tool was PowerPoint presentations of lecture outlines and other course material. Thus, further research is needed to examine the usefulness of this technological tool for online teaching.

The students primarily perceived the Discussion Board as an opportunity for them to learn and share information with other students on the web-based course. In the future, the instructor might consider assigning each student the responsibility of serving as a facilitator for a specific forum on the Discussion Board. This could be a creative way to weave opportunities for learner-learner interactions into the web-based course.

More than a majority of the students perceived the video clips to be useful in serving as a reminder about assignments and course requirements and for providing a sense of connectedness to the instructor. However, creating multi-media presentations, such as a video clip, can be a very frustrating endeavor for the instructor. Stafford and Namorato (1998) attest to the fact that the learning curve for using this technology is fairly steep and very specific. Creating the presentations requires a major commitment of time, as well as persistence to tolerate the inevitable glitches in capturing, editing, and making these clips.

Students expressed more satisfaction with the level of instructor-learner interaction than with the level of learner-learner interaction. This is not a surprising finding considering that students interacted more with the instructor around completing course requirements and maneuvering through cyberspace. In fact, the students reported that they primarily sought technical assistance for completing the web-based course from the instructor. Future research is needed, however, to examine the quality of the relationships formed between instructors and students when using electronic pedagogy as the instructional method.

The two major assignments, the social policy analysis and the electronic policy advocacy, were perceived to be useful by the students in increasing their knowledge base related to policy practice. Encouraging students to use electronic communications in influencing or contacting stakeholders to effect policy change is supported by Miller-Cribbs and Chadiha (1998) and by Fitzgerald and McNutt (1999).

Almost a fourth of the students expressed a desire for more personal interactions with the instructor. This again affirms the importance of weaving interactivity in the virtual classroom. Faux and Black-Hughes (2000) contend that using the Internet as an instructional tool must take into account the students' needs for interaction with the instructor.

Of significance is the finding that females were more likely to ask for technical assistance than were their male counterparts. Likewise, in Roberts-DeGennaro and Clapp's (2002) study, males reported to be more comfortable with learning about and using computers, particularly in regards to liking computers.

The most positive statement regarding the web-based course was the finding that over 90% of the students would take another online course and would also recommend this specific course to another student.

Overall, the course evaluation ratings indicate that the students enjoyed learning as much through the virtual classroom of a web-based course as through a traditional on-campus classroom.

IMPLICATIONS FOR WEB-BASED TEACHING IN SOCIAL WORK EDUCATION

The integration of technological tools for weaving interactivity into a web-based course is critical to the effectiveness of a virtual classroom. Key to the online learning process are the interactions among the students, the interactions between the instructor and the students, and the collaborative learning process that results from these interactions.

Moore (1989) contends that the learner-learner interaction is probably the most challenging type of interaction to implement in distance education. Online discussions help to promote a sense that there are real people that the students are interacting with when they communicate through the cyberspace of a virtual classroom. Knowlton, Knowlton, and Davis (2000) support the use of online discussions as students become part of an educational cyber-community of learners rather than feeling alone in the educational process. Palloff and Pratt (1999) suggest that a web of learning is created through the use of online discussions. Students are not only responsible for logging on to the web-based course, but are expected to contribute to the learning process by posting their thoughts and ideas, for example, to a forum on a Discussion Board.

A commonly used computer-based teaching tool is the construction of PowerPoint presentations. More creative approaches are needed in developing these presentations. Stocks and Freddolino (1998) suggest that a "thought problem" link could be inserted into these presentations. For example, a controversial question could be posed to students in the online PowerPoint lecture notes, which is then followed by a link to a listserv discussion list. Participation in this listserv might encourage more learner-learner and learner-instructor interaction.

The availability of training to support educational plans for building competencies in teaching through the virtual classroom is paramount to the success of online learning. This should include training on the use of technology for course development and on the methodology of electronic pedagogy. The availability of top-of-the-line software and up-to-date hardware is critical to constructing a web-based course. Both the instructor and the students must have access to technical support through the institution. In addition, adequate support has to be provided to these instructors by the administration at all levels within the university.

In online teaching, the instructor is predominantly represented by the textual content of the course, rather than the personality of the instructor. Thus, seasoned instructors should be the dominant course developers for online programs since they understand the nature of the student population and the curriculum content for the courses, including competencies for professional social work practice.

Sandell and Hayes (2002) recently raised the question whether institutions of higher education are ready to champion and pay for course development, technological support, and the new creative synergies that are needed to make electronic courses effective, as well as to support research to investigate the effectiveness of electronic pedagogy. Schools of social work that do not have access to cutting edge technology in planning, constructing, and delivering web-based, or even web-assisted, courses might find their programs on the downside of the digital divide.

REFERENCES

Anderson, T., & Garrison, D. R. (1998). Learning in a networked world: New roles and responsibilities. In C. Campbell Gibson (Ed.), *Distance learners in higher education: Institutional responses for quality outcomes* (pp. 97-112). Madison, WI: Atwood Publishing.

Crook, W., & Brady, M. (1998). Computer-assisted instruction in the classroom: Using a web shell. In F. Raymond, L. Ginsberg, & D. Gohagan (Eds.), *Information technologies: Teaching to use–Using to teach* (pp. 193-208). New York: The Haworth Press, Inc.

Faux, T., & Black-Hughes, C. (2000). A comparison of using the Internet versus lectures to teach social work history. *Research on Social Work Practice, 10* (4), 454-466.

Fitzgerald, E., & McNutt, J. (1999). Electronic advocacy in policy practice: A framework for teaching technologically based practice. *Journal of Social Work Education, 35* (3), 331-341.

Garrison, D. (1989). *Understanding distance education: A framework for the future*. New York: Routledge.

Graves, W. (2000). The dot.xxx challenge to higher education. *Syllabus, 13* (10), 30, 32, 34, & 36.

Hantula, D. (1998). The virtual industrial/organizational psychology class: Learning and teaching in cyberspace in three iterations. *Behavior Research Methods, Instruments, & Computers, 30* (2), 205-216.

Harrington, D. (1999). Teaching statistics: A comparison of traditional classroom and programmed instruction/distance learning approaches. *Journal of Social Work Education, 35* (3), 343-352.

Hodes, C. (1997-98). Developing a rationale for technology integration. *Journal of Educational Technology Systems, 26* (3), 225-234.

Knowles, A. (2001). Implementing web-based learning: Evaluation results from a mental health course. In J. Miller-Cribbs (Ed.), *New advances in technology for social work education and practice* (pp. 171-187). New York: The Haworth Press, Inc.

Knowlton, D., Knowlton, H., & Davis, C. (2000). The whys and hows of online discussion. *Syllabus, 13* (10), 54-56, 58.

Miller-Cribbs, J., & Chadiha, L. (1998). Integrating the Internet in a human diversity course. In F. Raymond, L. Ginsberg, & D. Gohagan (Eds.), *Information technologies: Teaching to use–Using to teach* (pp. 97-108). New York: The Haworth Press, Inc.

Moore, M. (1989). Three types of interaction. In M. Moore & G. C. Clark (Eds.), *Readings in principles of distance education* (pp. 100-105). University Park, PA: American Center for the Study of Distance Education.

Palloff, R., & Pratt, K. (1999). *Building learning communities in cyberspace: Effective strategies for the online classroom.* San Francisco: Jossey-Bass.

Raymond, F., Ginsberg, L., & Gohagan, D. (1998). Introduction. In F. Raymond, L. Ginsberg & D. Gohagan (Eds.), *Information technologies: Teaching to use–Using to teach* (pp. 1-5). New York: The Haworth Press, Inc.

Raymond, F., & Pike, C. (1997). Social work education: Electronic technologies. In R. Edwards (Ed.), *Encyclopedia of social work, 19th edition, 1997 supplement* (pp. 281-299). Washington DC: National Association of Social Workers Press.

Roberts-DeGennaro, M. (2002). Constructing and implementing a web-based graduate social policy course: A pilot test in cyberspace. *Social Policy Journal, 1* (2), 73-90.

Roberts-DeGennaro, M., & Clapp, J. D. (2002). *Comparative study of a web-based and on-campus social policy course: Attitudes toward learning about and using computers.* Manuscript submitted for publication, School of Social Work, San Diego State University.

Royse, D. (2000). Teaching research online: A process evaluation. *Journal of Teaching in Social Work, 20* (1/2), 145-158.

Sandell, K., & Hayes, S. (2002). The web's impact on social work education: Opportunities, challenges, and future directions. *Journal of Social Work Education, 38* (1), 85-99.

Sarnoff, S. (2001). Ensuring that course websites are ADA compliant. In J. Miller-Cribbs (Ed.), *New advances in technology for social work education and practice* (pp. 189-201). New York: The Haworth Press, Inc.

Schoech, D. (2000). Teaching over the Internet: Results of one doctoral course. *Research on Social Work Practice, 10* (4), 467-486.

Seaberg, J. (1999). *The virtual classroom, asynchronous teaching via the Internet.* Retrieved December 3, 2001, from: http://www.people.vcu.edu/~jseaberg/virtual_classroom.htm

Seaberg, J. (2001). *Use of the Internet and other teaching tools in graduate social work education.* Retrieved December 3, 2001, from: http://www.people.vcu.edu/~jseaberg/teaching_survey.htm

Siegel, E., Jennings, J., Conklin, J., & Napoletano-Flynn, S. (1998). Distance learning in social work education: Results and implications of a national study. *Journal of Social Work Education, 34,* 71-80.

Sieppert, J., & Krysik, J. (1996). Computer-based testing in social work education: A preliminary exploration. *Computers in Human Services, 13* (1), 43-61.

Sonwalkar, N. (2001). The sharp edge of the cube: Pedagogically driven instructional design for online education. *Syllabus, 15* (5), 12-14, & 16.

Stafford, J., & Namorato, M. (1998). Multi-media computer technology in the classroom. In F. Raymond, L. Ginsberg, & D. Gohagan (Eds.), *Information technologies: Teaching to use–Using to teach* (pp. 185-191). New York: The Haworth Press, Inc.

Stocks, J., & Freddolino, P. (1998). Evaluation of a World Wide Web-based graduate social work research methods course. In F. Raymond, L. Ginsberg, & D. Gohagan (Eds.), *Information technologies: Teaching to use–Using to teach* (pp. 51-69). New York: The Haworth Press, Inc.

Stocks, J., & Freddolino, P. (2000). Enhancing computer-mediated teaching through interactivity: The second iteration of a World Wide Web-based graduate social work course. *Research on Social Work Practice, 10* (4), 505-518.

W3C (1999). *Web content accessibility guidelines 1.0.* Retrieved March 19, 2002, from: http://www.w3.org/TR/WAI-WEBCONTENT/

Zhang, P. (1998). A case study on technology use in distance learning. *Journal of Research on Computing in Education, 30* (4), 398-416.

PART II

PART

The Transition from Traditional Teaching to Web-Assisted Technology

Andy J. Frey

Anna C. Faul

SUMMARY. This research note presents a conceptual model for understanding how students embrace technology, briefly presents results of a pilot study supporting this conceptualization, and makes suggestions for web-assisted teaching and research. The conceptual framework helps the reader understand how instructors' "Marketing strategies" may need to change over the course of the semester to generate maximum acceptance of, and satisfaction with, high-tech classrooms. The conceptual framework is illustrated with data collected during a pilot study involving two web-assisted graduate foundation research courses at the Kent School of Social Work, University of Louisville. Students enrolled for two web-assisted research courses without knowing that web-assisted technology would be used in the course. The students' attitudes towards

---

Andy J. Frey, PhD, Assistant Professor, and Anna C. Faul, PhD, Assistant Professor, are affiliated with the Kent School of Social Work, University of Louisville, Louisville, KY.

Address correspondence to: Andy J. Frey, PhD, Kent School of Social Work, University of Louisville, Louisville, KY 40292 (E-mail: ajfrey0l@louisville.edu).

The authors are not listed in order of contribution to this study. The contribution was of equal value.

[Haworth co-indexing entry note]: "The Tansition from Traditional Teaching to Web-Assisted Technology." Frey, Andy J., and Anna C. Faul. Co-published simultaneously in *Journal of Teaching in Social Work* (The Haworth Social Work Practice Press, an imprint of The Haworth Press, Inc.) Vol. 25, No. 1/2, 2005, pp. 91-101; and: *Technology in Social Work Education and Curriculum: The High Tech, High Touch Social Work Educator* (ed: Richard L. Beaulaurier, and Martha Haffey) The Haworth Social Work Practice Press, an imprint of The Haworth Press, Inc., 2005, pp. 91-101. Single or multiple copies of this article are available for a fee from The Haworth Document Delivery Service [1-800-HAWORTH, 9:00 a.m. - 5:00 p.m. (EST). E-mail address: docdelivery@haworthpress.com].

computers, their ability to access computers, as well as their skill levels in using computers were assessed. Suggestions and challenges for web-assisted teaching and research are provided based on the conceptual framework and results from the pilot study. *[Article copies available for a fee from The Haworth Document Delivery Service: 1-800-HAWORTH. E-mail address: <docdelivery@haworthpress.com> Website: <http://www.HaworthPress.com> © 2005 by The Haworth Press, Inc. All rights reserved.]*

KEYWORDS. Web-assisted teaching, distance education, social work education, attitudes toward computers, attitudes research

The use of technology is revolutionizing university education for both faculty and students, yet the benefits and drawbacks are different for each. There is a wide range of experiences among students and faculty members, and understanding the process by which each embraces or rejects technology is critical for schools interested in increasing the use of technology in instruction. Until recently, allowing students to enroll in web-assisted courses without first informing them of the technology to be used may have been considered unethical, and still may be perceived as unfair by students who have negative attitudes towards technology, or those for whom computer access is not readily available. Nonetheless, instructors are increasingly relying on technology, and often a minimum level of technological expertise is an unstated prerequisite for the course. For example, some students may be required to log on to the web, use e-mail, or conduct basic web searches even though the course was not advertised as a technology intensive course. Despite much enthusiasm for new technology, little data is available for instructors to make data-based decisions concerning which strategies to use. Additionally, little is known about student experiences with web-assisted technology. If social work education is to take web-assisted instruction seriously, the profession must begin to generate a research base that supports its use.

This research note presents a conceptual model for understanding how students adapt to web-assisted technology and briefly presents results of a pilot study supporting the model. The note concludes by making suggestions for web-assisted teaching and research.

THE ADAPTATION OF WEB-ASSISTED TECHNOLOGY

The most compelling framework to understand how consumers embrace technology comes from business. Moore's (1999) Business Week bestseller, *Inside the tornado: Marketing strategies from Silicon Valley's cutting edge,* analyzes the strategies of high-tech companies that have thrived, and those that have failed. The lessons learned, however, apply not only to high-tech companies, but to all innovations or new products or services that require the consumer and the marketplace to dramatically change their behavior, with the promise of achieving equally dramatic new benefits.

Moore (1999) identifies five groups of constituencies: technology enthusiasts, visionaries, pragmatists, conservatives, and skeptics. According to the framework, technology enthusiasts and visionaries are those who want to use innovation even if the benefits have not been firmly established. The pragmatists do not love technology for its own sake, but believe in evolution, and will make the transition once a proven track record exists. The conservatives are not passionate about technology in general, and undertake such changes under duress; they are price sensitive and demanding. Skeptics are eternal critics, are not likely to convert, and are to be avoided, according to Moore.

Based on these profiles, Moore (1999) suggests that whenever innovative products are introduced into the marketplace they receive a warm welcome from technology enthusiasts and visionaries, but then will fall into the *chasm,* a lag in eagerness for the product as the pragmatists wait for the product to be complete. Pragmatists then watch carefully as the technology enthusiasts and visionaries test the product to see how they might benefit. Moore's (1999) premise in the book is that the only way to cross the chasm, or reach the mainstream market, is to gain a hold of a niche market, putting all your effort on a narrowly focused area. During this stage of product evolution, customer service is the primary goal. After the chasm is crossed, the marketing strategy must shift from a focus on customer service to high production at any cost.

This conceptualization can inform the use of web-assisted technology in several respects. First, it provides a framework for instructors to understand where students are coming from, and what students will expect to occur before they are satisfied with innovative teaching strategies relying on technology. It also helps instructors to think about how web-assisted strategies can be introduced, or marketed, to students.

PILOT STUDY

Blackboard, a course authoring software package, provides an excellent opportunity for faculty and students to become familiar with new web-assisted courses. The software creates the opportunity for aspects of course delivery to be online in a user-friendly, flexible environment. Palloff and Pratt (2001) rate Blackboard as one of the few course authoring software systems that is functional–simple to operate for both faculty and students, user-friendly, visually appealing, and easy to navigate. As instructors continue to rely on web-assisted instruction, it is important to determine not only how students who would voluntarily enroll in a course using web-assisted technology experience the course, but also how those who would not choose this option respond to technology.

The research course that was transformed for this pilot study into a web-assisted technology course has been a well-designed course for many years. The authors redesigned this course into a web-assisted course by rethinking the learning outcomes, the methods of instruction, the course content and the assessment of student performance.

With the help of the Blackboard interface the syllabus was posted on-line and faculty information was provided on the instructors with a specific invitation to students to reach them any time via e-mail. Specific student tools were made available, for example the opportunity to create homepages in order to become familiar with fellow classmates, the electronic submission of assignments in the "digital drop box," the ability to access their grades on-line, the option to send e-mail to any or all of the students in their class, the opportunity to start their own discussion groups, and access to on-line resource links. Detailed session outlines were posted for each of the 10 contact sessions that included the purpose of the session, topics to be covered, assignments due, required readings, and on-line session notes that could be printed before class. In-class discussions centered on the readings and the session notes as well as class assignments. Formal lecturing was restricted and the main emphasis in class was on interaction regarding the session content posted on the web. On-line quizzes were designed and posted for each session to help students assess their own progress in the mastery of the research content taught in each session. The assignments were provided in an on-line format, where students were able to download the assignment from the web, complete it on-line, and submit it electronically.

Methods

The study consisted of an evaluation of two web-assisted courses with the authors as instructors; both courses were taught in the summer of 2001 at the Kent School of Social Work, University of Louisville.

Students did not know before they signed up for the course that the course would be a web-assisted course. The evaluation was done to gain an understanding of how students embrace a course that utilizes a relatively high degree of web-assisted instruction, and to determine if any support could be garnered for Moore's (1999) conceptual framework suggesting a developmental component to the adoption of web-assisted strategies.

Participants. Thirty-two students enrolled for the two research methods courses. Seven of the students were male and 25 were female. Their age ranged between 25 and 55, with mean ages of 35.45 (SD = 9.12). Twenty-seven of the students were Euro-American, four were African-American, and one was Native American.

Measures. Students completed a background questionnaire, a Computer Access Questionnaire (CAQ) and a Computer Attitude Scale (CAS) during the first class session. The CAQ is designed by the SNOW Project Team (2000) as a 17-item instrument focusing on the accessibility of computers, modems, and the Internet to students. The CAS is a 30-item, rapid assessment instrument developed by Lloyd and Gressard (1984). It is designed to measure the respondent's comfort with computers. Respondents are asked to indicate their level of agreement with statements on a seven-point Likert Scale. Example items include: computers do not scare me at all; I would like working with computers; and generally, I would feel OK about trying a new problem on the computer. Higher scores indicate greater comfort.

The students were asked at the completion of the course to assess the perceived value of the different web technology that was used. The Value Rating Checklist of Web-Assisted Technology (VRCWAT) was compiled by the researchers and consists of 19 questions. The VRC WAT was created by the authors for the purpose of this study. Personal knowledge and the available literature on web-assisted instruction helped generate items for the VRCWAT. The three authors have seven years combined experience using Blackboard, Eduprise, and WebCT as course authoring software. The literature base also helped to provide examples of various strategies that have been attributed to increased knowledge and positive experiences for students enrolled in courses utilizing technology (Flynn, 1990; Maki, Maki, Patterson, & Whittaker, 2000; Stocks & Freddolino, 1998; Stocks & Freddolino, 2000; Thurston, Denning, & Verschelden, 1996). The VRCWAT is not believed to be a unidimensional construct, but a checklist of the web-assisted technology strategies used in the course. Students were asked to indicate their perceived value of each of the 18 different web-assisted strategies. Scores were rated on an anchored scale ranging between 1 and 7, with 1 indicating *no value at all* and 7 indicating *very valuable*. If the instructor did not use a specific strategy, the students were asked to check the *not applicable* option.

Procedure and Results

Students arrived at the two different classes without any knowledge that they would make use of web-assisted technology. The research study was introduced to the students. All students in the web-assisted classes consented to the research and completed the background questionnaire, the CAQ and the CAS. All students completed open-ended evaluation sheets following each session and e-mailed their instructor weekly. At the end of the course the students completed the VRCWAT.

The results of the CAS indicated that there was a wide range of attitudes towards computers among the students at the beginning of the course. The scores on the CAS could range between 30 and 210 with higher scores indicating more positive attitudes. The scores for the 32 students ranged from 55 to 210, representing a wide distribution of the attitudes among students.

Students' proficiency with computers was assessed using three single-item indicators from the CAQ relating to comfort level with computers, level of computer ability, and computer keyboard skills. The indicators were measured on a Likert Scale that ranged from 1 to 7, with a higher score indicating greater proficiency. Students also had a wide distribution of scores for these three variables. Single items regarding access to computers and the Internet on the CAQ suggested students enrolled in graduate school have reasonable access to computers and the Internet. All 32 students in the study had access to a computer, with 25 of the students having computers at home. Six had access to a computer only at work, and one had access to a computer only on campus. All of the students had access to the Internet.

Student e-mails throughout the semester provided some preliminary support for the applicability of Moore's (1999) conceptual framework concerning the student adoption of web-assisted technology strategies. During the first session, the students were introduced to the syllabus by means of PowerPoint slide printouts that provided a summary of the course syllabus. Students were very apprehensive about not receiving the full syllabus in hard copy form. The students with negative attitudes towards computers and low proficiency in the use of computers had tremendous fears that they would not be able to succeed in class due to their technological skill.

The week after the first session numerous e-mails were received by the instructors concerning access to the site. Students also expressed discontent with the syllabus, which was not handed out in class. One of the students commented: *"At this moment I would like to say that the conventional syllabus seems to be much easier to deal with than the web thing. And this is from a person that loves the computer, e-mail, and the Internet. It feels like too much work to figure out what the work really is."* For these students, the instructors tried to validate concerns, and be as supportive as possible. It was important to be available for phone calls during the first few weeks.

After the first assignment, students started to embrace the web-assisted technology. Specifically, the guidance they received from the instructors, the quick feedback, the availability of the grades before the next class, and the ease in which they could submit their assignments changed some of the attitudes of the students. One student commented, *"Since I complained about the Internet aspect of this course last week let me say something positive this week. I do think it is convenient to be able to turn in and receive papers through the web. I also enjoy being able to receive my grade in this manner and to see my standing in the course compared to the class average. Your guiding us through this process, reminding us about projects and the discussion board is also a great help. Thanks!!"*

Students with less proficiency in the use of web-assisted technology were frightened at first, but they started to overcome their fears. Some of the weekly feedback indicated their progress: *"I am getting the hang of using the computer program, but still get frustrated at times." "I actually got the survey and questions to print!! I am so happy. Thanks for the help!!"* As the course developed, students started to use most of the technology effectively and with confidence. The students with positive attitudes and skills towards computers at the beginning of the course had no problems throughout the course, adapted to the technology, and used it to their advantage. After the students overcame their original fears and became more accustomed to the web-assisted technology, a normal course process developed. The strategy of instructors changed at this time; rather than focus on the technological support for the two or three skeptics, efforts were directed at reviewing and returning assignments rapidly. In this sense, the strategy was reversed from customer service to production. The content of the e-mails became more directed towards course content and less on how to use the Blackboard site. The students learned to appreciate the value of the new technology, and started to use it to their own advantage.

Not surprisingly, there were a few students who just could not adapt to the web-assisted technology. One student lost her motivation for the course, and after late submissions on two assignments, a discussion ensued where she stated her poor performance in the course was related to the technology. While several other students expressed frustration initially, the two web-assisted courses ended with only one student who maintained the web-assisted strategies used were unfair and discriminatory.

The results of the Value Rating Scale of Web-Assisted Technology (VRCWAT) showed that the posting of on-line lecture notes, e-mail communication with students, posting of on-line grades, on-line feedback regarding assignments and detailed assignment instructions on-line were viewed as the web-assisted techniques that were most helpful to student learning. The availability of home pages to post personal information and on-line discussion groups were reported as the least effective.

SUGGESTIONS AND CHALLENGES
FOR WEB-ASSISTED TEACHING

Teachers utilizing web-assisted technology are likely to benefit from Moore's (1999) advice to market technology to students differently over the course of the semester. During the first few weeks of the course, instructors can appeal to the technology enthusiasts so they will educate the visionaries. Instructors next can engage and support the visionaries, hoping they will convince the pragmatists of the benefits of web-assisted strategies. Ultimately, teachers hope the pragmatists will convince the conservatives that the use of technology is worth their while. This process can be expedited by facilitating conversations in the class among early technology users.

Teachers should be mindful that a large range of attitudes towards computers and proficiency with computers still exist among social work students. However, this should not limit their use of technology in the classroom, only their approach to students. What is, however, encouraging, is that this pilot study suggests it may be safe to assume that students will have access to the technology required to navigate a course that relies heavily on computer-assisted technology.

The process evaluation demonstrates that even if all students have access to the web, there may be a small percentage of students who resist the movement towards technology, and a very small percentage who never embrace it, or worse, believe it compromises their learning experience. On the other hand, most students support the use of technology from the beginning, and many who initially raise concerns recognize the advantages by the conclusion of the semester. If instructors are going to use web-assisted technology extensively in courses where enrolling students are not made aware of the technology requirements, they may want to identify alternative placement options or highlight what is required in the way of technology early on so students who strongly oppose the use of technology can make alternative plans.

The results of the VRCWAT showed that students value the interaction with their instructor via web-assisted technology. They also valued immediate feedback related to assignments and grades. All these aspects are crucial to secure a successful learning experience. However, the fact that the participants did not care for the personalized homepages and the on-line discussion groups is a problem. The aspect of collaboration between classmates via the web should be developed further if mixed mode or web-based courses are developed for social work courses. The cooperation among students is an important variable in the success of courses and cannot be ignored (Palloff & Pratt, 2001).

CHALLENGES AND ISSUES
FOR WEB-ASSISTED TECHNOLOGY RESEARCH

Much of the research in the area of web technology relates to satisfaction. However, measures of satisfaction are extremely limited, and do not inform instructors what is potentially valuable and what is not. Moore's conceptualization and the findings for this pilot study can be a guide for future research relating to web-assisted technology. There are several questions that would benefit social work education if conducted with large, representative, samples. For example, *what specific web-assisted strategies are the most and least helpful to students? Do student value perceptions differ based on their learning style, ability to access computers, keyboarding skills, or their attitude towards computers? Are value perceptions similar for students in different types of courses or for students who commute versus those who live locally?* Documenting the process from students' perspectives would also be valuable to determine the differences between students who embrace the technology and those who do not. Another area of interest involves the process by which instructors adapt to web-assisted techniques. *How many courses do instructors have to conduct before they experience the bene-*

fits of web-assisted technology? What level of support is required to have positive experiences?

Concerning methodology, it is important to recruit a sample that is representative of larger groups of social work students. One challenge facing researchers examining the value of web-assisted technology is to control for the instructor variable. Like satisfaction, it is difficult to know if students are reporting on the value of the web-assisted strategy or to the extent to which they like their instructor. Another challenge is keeping up-to-date with the rapidly changing technology strategies available to instructors. It seems the number of strategies is growing faster than our ability to research them.

CONCLUSION

Similar to the talk of managed care a decade or so ago, the question is not whether or not the transition to web-assisted technology will take place, but how fast–and will we be prepared when it does. Moore's (1999) lessons learned from the high-tech industry are extremely helpful in understanding how students will embrace instructional technology, and how instructors can better market technology to enhance students' acceptability of the strategies. This pilot study lends initial support for the presence of early adopters, visionaries, pragmatists, conservatives and skeptics within our student population. Additionally, the pilot study generated several research questions that are worthy of investigation, and outlines some of the challenges likely to be encountered by those who seek answers to them.

REFERENCES

Flynn, J. P. (1990). Using the computer to teach and learn social policy: A report from the classroom and the field. *Computers in Human Services, 7*(3-4), 199-209.

Lloyd, B. H., & Gressard, C. P. (1984). Reliability and factorial validity of computer attitude scales. *Educational and Psychological Measurement, 44*, 501-505.

Maki, R. H., Maki, W. S., Patterson, M., & Whittaker, P. D. (2000). Evaluation of a web-based introductory psychology course: I. Learning and satisfaction in on-line versus lecture courses. *Behavior Research Methods, Instruments, and Computers, 32*(2), 230-239.

Moore, G. A. (1999). *Inside the tornado: Marketing strategies from Silicon Valley's cutting edge.* New York, NY: HarperCollins Publishers.

Palloff, R. M., & Pratt, K. (2001). *Lessons from the cyberspace classroom. The realities of online teaching.* San Francisco: Jossey-Bass.

SNOW Project Team (2000). *Inclusion in an electronic classroom.* Available: *http://snow.utoronto.ca/initiatives/*

Stocks, J. T., & Freddolino, P. P. (1998). Evaluation of a worldwide web-based graduate social work research methods course. *Computers in Human Services, 15*(2/3), 51-69.

Stocks, J. T., & Freddolino, P. P. (2000). Enhancing computer-mediated teaching through interactivity: The second iteration of a worldwide web-based graduate social work course. *Research on Social Work Practice, 10*(4), 505-518.

Thurston, L. P., Denning, J., & Verschelden, C. (1996). Using interactive multimedia to address rural social work education needs. In E. T. Reck (Ed.), *Tulane studies in social welfare.* New Orleans, LA: Tulane School of Social Work.

An Evaluation of On-Line,
Interactive Tutorials
Designed to Teach Practice Concepts

Brett A. Seabury

SUMMARY. This paper presents an evaluation of two on-line-based programs designed to teach practice skills. One program teaches crisis intervention and the other teaches suicide assessment. The evaluation of the use of these programs compares outcomes for two groups of students, one using the interactive program outside a class context and the other using the program within the class. Additionally, the evaluation examines results of learning about crisis of these two groups in comparison to a group of students who did not use the programs. Outcomes suggest advantages in using interactive on-line tutorials in efficiency and objectivity. This paper hopes to encourage other faculty to develop similar programs that simulate various elements of social work practice. *[Article copies available for a fee from The Haworth Document Delivery Service: 1-800-HAWORTH. E-mail address: <docdelivery@haworthpress. com> Website: <http://www.HaworthPress.com> © 2005 by The Haworth Press, Inc. All rights reserved.]*

Brett A. Seabury, DSW, ACSW, is Associate Professor, School of Social Work, University of Michigan, 1080 South University, Ann Arbor, MI 48109-1106 (E-mail: bseabury@umich.edu).

[Haworth co-indexing entry note]: "An Evaluation of On-Line, Interactive Tutorials Designed to Teach Practice Concepts." Seabury, Brett A. Co-published simultaneously in *Journal of Teaching in Social Work* (The Haworth Social Work Practice Press, an imprint of The Haworth Press, Inc.) Vol. 25, No. 1/2, 2005, pp. 103-115; and: *Technology in Social Work Education and Curriculum: The High Tech, High Touch Social Work Educator* (ed: Richard L. Beaulaurier, and Martha Haffey) The Haworth Social Work Practice Press, an imprint of The Haworth Press, Inc., 2005, pp. 103-115. Single or multiple copies of this article are available for a fee from The Haworth Document Delivery Service [1-800-HAWORTH, 9:00 a.m. - 5:00 p.m. (EST). E-mail address: docdelivery@haworthpress.com].

Digital Object Identifier: 10.1300/J067v25n01_07   *103*

KEYWORDS. Distance education, crisis intervention, suicide assessment, computer programs, social work education, interactive video simulations

Computer-assisted instruction and interactive video have been employed in many fields as a training tool. Pilots and astronauts are trained on simulators before they ever fly the real thing. Medical students are trained with simulated scenarios in order to learn medical protocols (http://www.osl.u-net.com/m410.htm–website last accessed on 11/22/02). The nursing profession uses interactive video programs to teach nursing students various diagnostic techniques (Lambrecht, 1991; http://products.fitne.net/catalog/toc.asp–website last accessed on 11/22/02). Educational research has generally demonstrated the efficacy of interactive video as a training strategy (McNeil & Nelson, 1991), and some educators have even asserted that interactive tutorials are superior to didactic classroom instruction when it comes to teaching basic skills (Bosco & Wagner, 1988).

Over the past decade, various kinds of computer-based programs have been developed in social work education that attempt to teach practice skills (Goldberg & Middleman, 1987; Maple, Kleinsmith, & Kleinsmith, 1991). A handful of interactive video disc (IVD) programs have appeared in social work (Carlson, Bogen, & Pettit, 1989; Falk, Shepard, Campbell, & Maypole, 1992; Maple, 1994; Maypole, 1991; Resnick, 1994; Seabury, 1993). Recently, commercial CD-ROM programs have emerged that are designed to teach various direct practice skills (Sevel, Cummins, & Madrigal, 1999; Haney & Leibsohn, 1999; Haney & Leibsohn, 2001).

This paper will focus on two interactive, on-line programs that were designed by this author to teach students how to apply practice concepts to a video simulation. These programs have been evaluated from three perspectives: (1) the reactions and perceptions of students completing these on-line tutorial programs; (2) the ability of students to pass an outcome measure (i.e., quiz) after completing these tutorials; and (3) a comparison of three classes of social work students. One class completed the interactive tutorial on crisis intervention, another class experienced a classroom presentation on crisis interventions, and a third class completed the outcome measure before receiving training in crisis intervention.

DESCRIPTION OF PROGRAMS

The first program ("Crisis Counseling: I Am Chipper!") teaches students how to apply crisis concepts to an individual client in active crisis. The second program ("Suicide Prevention Simulation: Rube Farmer") teaches students how to apply risk factors to a depressed client with suicidal ideation. These programs are not designed to teach interviewing skills, as are the commercial CD-ROM programs, but instead are designed to teach students how to assess and intervene in practice situations involving crisis and suicide. These tutorial programs have five parts: (1) an interactive, PowerPoint™ tutorial which covers basic principles and concepts; (2) an interactive video simulation which simulates a practice experience; (3) a follow-up quiz which requires students to connect concepts from the tutorial to the video simulation; (4) an online evaluation; and (5) a selected bibliography.

These programs are designed as self-instructional tutorials, which can be completed in about two hours by a conscientious student, or they can be used in a classroom setting with a computer-assisted projection system. These programs are available in CD-ROM format and can be played on a Pentium II platform or higher with CD-ROM player and RealMedia™ player installed. They can also be downloaded from the Internet–i.e., the tutorial as an Acrobat Reader PDF file and the video simulation streamed as RealMedia™ files. In both the CD-ROM form and the Internet versions, the quiz and evaluation sections are on-line and sent directly back to this author as an e-mail message (see Figure 1).

The Crisis program is the longer of the two and covers key concepts in crisis assessment and intervention such as stressful conditions, hazardous events, vulnerable state, precipitating factor, active crisis, and intervention strategies (Seabury, 2004). The video simulation is about a graduating student, Chipper, who is coping with the stressors of completing course assignments, looking for a job after graduation, as well as preparing for impending parenthood. The crisis video simulates an interview with this client, and contains case information that reflects all of the concepts presented in the tutorial. The quiz requires the student to connect crisis concepts to the video simulation–e.g., what was the precipitant that pushed "Chipper" into active crisis?

The Suicide Assessment program presents key concepts in assessing the lethality of suicide in a client–such as right-to-die issues, cultural factors, risk factors, assessment scales, suicide prevention, and myths about suicide. When the student begins the video simulation with Rube, who is portrayed as an elderly, white, rural, working-class farmer, the

FIGURE 1. Crisis Intervention Tutorial

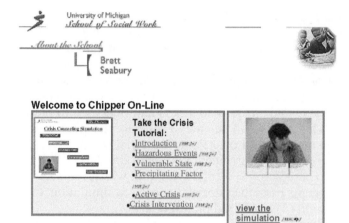

student must identify her/himself using the basic identity issues of gender and ethnicity. This identification triggers different beginnings, and Rube "gives the student a hard time" about whether the student will be able to understand his troubles. The student must cope with this reluctance to cooperate on Rube's part before moving into the interview to discover what is going on in his life situation. It is suggested that students interview Rube at least twice before completing the quiz in order to get the information to judge how seriously suicidal he is. The quiz requires the student to connect suicide concepts to Rube's life situation, to explain the sources of Rube's reluctance to cooperate in the interview, and to decide and rationalize whether he needs emergency hospitalization.

EVALUATION OF ON-LINE TUTORIALS

These two programs were employed in a foundation micro methods course as one of several optional grading exercises. The crisis program has been available to students on-line for five semesters, and the suicide program has been available for three semesters. Sixty-six students completed the crisis tutorial and all but two passed the on-line quiz. Thirty-six students completed the suicide tutorial and all passed the on-line quiz. In order to get credit for completing the tutorial, students had to pass the quiz with an 85% or better accuracy level. If the on-line quiz is viewed as one kind of outcome measure, then it is clear that all but two of the 102 students who completed both tutorial and the interactive interviews were able to apply crisis concepts and suicide concepts to the simulated interviews.[1]

Students who completed these on-line tutorials were also asked to complete anonymously and voluntarily a brief evaluation of their perceptions of these two programs as educational experiences. The number of students completing these evaluations (N = 24 for the crisis tutorial and N = 7 for the suicide tutorial) is small, but some trends are evident in these data. The trends are consistent with other student evaluations of interactive video tutorials (Seabury & Maple, 1993).

For those students who completed the evaluation of the on-line crisis tutorial, most students completed the program between one and two hours. Only three students did it in less than an hour. All (100%) of the students felt that they had learned about crisis theory, and 79% felt they had learned how to apply crisis concepts in practice. Almost all of the students (92%) felt the learning experience was enhanced by the interactive video; 96% were positive about this learning experience, and 84% felt the computer format facilitated the learning experience. Most of the students (88%) did not have trouble following the instructions and exercises in the program, but only a little over half (59%) felt the program was easier to complete than expected. When students were queried about this result, they explained that they had tried the crisis tutorial from home and could not get the video simulation to work because their modem connection was too slow. They had to complete the program in a University computer site.

Though the numbers of students who completed the evaluation of the suicide tutorial is very small, the trends are similar to the crisis evaluations. For those students who completed the evaluation of the suicide tutorial, completion of the on-line program took between 40 minutes and two hours. All of the students felt the learning experience was enhanced by the interactive video sequences, that it was a positive learning experience, and that the learning experience was facilitated by the computer format. Six of the seven students who completed the evaluation of the suicide program felt they had learned about suicide assessment and that they had learned how to apply suicide scales to practice.

The feedback from students who completed these two on-line programs in a micro method's course has been encouraging. Students were able to complete these two programs on-line and to pass ("B" or better) a quiz that covered the basic concepts in these programs. They were positive about the computer program and interactive simulations as learning experiences. The few students who completed both of these programs felt that the crisis program was more difficult to complete than the suicide assessment program. This may reflect the complexity and length of the crisis simulation because it is almost twice as long as the suicide simulation.

COMPARISON STUDY

A small study was designed that compared three groups of social work students. One class completed the interactive, computer-based tutorial on crisis (Tutorial), another class completed a more traditional classroom presentation on crisis theory (Classroom), and a third class completed the outcome measure before receiving classroom instruction in crisis theory (No Training). The design of this study was intended to demonstrate whether the two learning conditions were better than no training, and also to see if the interactive computer tutorial was as successful a learning condition as a more traditional classroom presentation of crisis theory.

The Sample

All subjects in the study were entering graduate social work students who were taking the introductory micro methods course. Three out of seven sections of this course participated in this study. Not all of the students in each of the classes completed the outcome measure. Participation was voluntary and some were absent on the day the presentation took place. In the tutorial group, 24 out of 28 students participated, in the classroom group, 19 out of 21 students participated, and in the no training group, 26 out of 28 students participated. The participation rates ranged from 86% in the tutorial group, to 90% in the classroom group, and to 92% in the control group.

Because these groups were not randomly assigned, demographic information about students was collected such as age, gender, ethnicity, years of prior experience in social work, and prior training in crisis theory. In order to see if there were significant differences between these three groups on the demographic and background variables, some of these variables were collapsed into groupings that eliminated cells with zeros so that Chi-square tests of significance could be performed. Chi-square demonstrated no significant difference between these three classes on background demographics (see Table 1).

In order to assure that the content of the classroom presentation was similar to the content of the interactive tutorial, the classroom presentation used the same slides and in the same order as the tutorial, both groups viewed the same video, and both groups had the chance to apply crisis concepts to the video. There were differences, however, between these two conditions. The tutorial was controlled by the computer, whereas the classroom presentation was controlled by the instructor. The students in the tutorial viewed the video as an interactive interview, whereas the students in the classroom viewed the video from beginning to end. The students in the tutorial took the quiz and received feedback from the computer about their answers, whereas the students in the

TABLE 1. Background Variables

	Tutorial	**Classroom**	**No Training**
NUMBER:	24	19*	27
GENDER:			
Female	19	15	19
Male	5	3	8
AGE:			
21-30	13 (54%)	12 (67%)	20 (74%)
31-40	4 (16%)	3 (17%)	3 (11%)
Over 40	7 (29%)	3 (17%)	4 (15%)
ETHNICITY:			
White	21 (88%)	12 (67%)	22 (81%)
Other[#]	3 (12%)	6 (33%)	5 (19%)
YRS EXPR IN HUM SVCS:			
0-1	7 (29%)	12 (63%)	11 (41%)
2-4	12 (50%)	4 (21%)	12 (44%)
5+	5 (21%)	3 (16%)	4 (15%)
PRIOR TRNG IN CRISIS:			
None	12 (50%)	14 (74%)	13 (48%)
Some	9 (38%)	4 (21%)	12 (44%)
Moderate+	3 (12%)	1 (5%)	2 (8%)

*One student in this class did not supply information on gender, age, and ethnicity.
[#]Other includes: Hispanic, African American, Asian American, Native American, and Foreign students.

classroom took the same quiz in the tutorial as a group and discussed their answers as a group. Both groups then completed the outcome measure.

In order to check on the quality of instruction, students were asked about their overall perceptions of the educational experience in both the tutorial and classroom. Students in both the tutorial group and the classroom group were overwhelmingly positive about the educational experience they received (see Tables 2 and 3). When these two groups are compared, the classroom group is more positive than the tutorial group.

The classroom group was more positive about the clarity of presentation, that examples clearly illustrated concepts, and that the method of instruction increased their interest in and knowledge of the subject matter.

Outcome Measure

The outcome measure for this study was a written crisis case from practice. Unlike the video simulation that involved a single individual (Chipper), this written case involved a family in active crisis. Students were instructed to go through this case and operationalize crisis concepts and to suggest specific interventions. For example, students were asked to identify precipitating factors, major stressors, and how members of the family coped during the vulnerable state, etc. This measure

TABLE 2. Students' Perception of Tutorial (N = 24)

Scale: Strongly Agree = 1, Agree = 2, Neutral = 3, Disagree = 4, Strongly Disagree = 5

	1	2	3	4	5	Mean
A. Crisis concepts were clearly presented.	12 50%	12 50%	0	0	0	1.5
B. The method of instruction increased my interest in this subject matter.	14 58%	8 33%	2 8%	0	0	1.5
C. The case examples clearly illustrated crisis concepts.	12 50%	12 50%	0	0	0	1.5
D. The method of instruction increased my knowledge of crisis theory.	8 33%	14 58%	2 8%	0	0	1.75
E. The method of instruction was interesting and helped me to pay attention to the presentation.	20 83%	3 13%	1 4%	0	0	1.21
F. I believe I can apply crisis theory in practice.	2 8%	17 71%	3 13%	2 8%	0	2.21

TABLE 3. Students' Perception of Classroom Presentation (N = 19)

Scale: Strongly Agree = 1, Agree = 2, Neutral = 3, Disagree = 4, Strongly Disagree = 5

	1	2	3	4	5	Mean
A. Crisis concepts were clearly presented.	16 84%	3 16%	0	0	0	1.16
B. The method of instruction increased my interest in this subject matter.	13 68%	6 32%	0	0	0	1.32
C. The case examples clearly illustrated crisis concepts.	13 68%	6 32%	0	0	0	1.32
D. The method of instruction increased my knowledge of crisis theory.	13 33%	6 58%	0 8%	0	0	1.32
E. The method of instruction was interesting and helped me to pay attention to the presentation.	15 79%	3 16%	1 5%	0	0	1.26
F. I believe I can apply crisis theory in practice.	7 8%	8 71%	4 13%	0 8%	0	1.84

also asked students to state specifically how they would apply various crisis intervention strategies–e.g., "How would you reconnect this family to existing supports?" and "How would you stay event-focused in this case?" In all there were 17 questions that students had to answer about this written case. All students (except those in the no training group) completed this measure immediately after they had completed the tutorial and class presentation on crisis theory.

Two experienced social work educators scored the outcome measure. Both scorers were "blind" and completed the scoring without knowing what cases were in what group. In order to check the inter-rater reliability of the scoring, a random subsample of 35 outcome measures was used to compare the two scorers. Even though this measure was viewed as a fairly objective test, we were surprised at the discrepancies of some item scores. The inter-rater reliability in this first round of scoring was (r = .75). The items with wide discrepancies were reviewed and discussed, and the differences between raters' scores were reduced to within two points. The remaining 34 cases in the sample were rescored which resulted in a higher inter-rater reliability level (r = .97).

Results

The results of this study supported the educational hypothesis proposed in the design. The tutorial group performed the best on the outcome measure and was significantly better than the no training group (Mann-Whitney U = 127.5, p = .000). The classroom group also performed significantly better on the outcome measure than the no training group (Mann-Whitney U = 121.5, p = .004) The classroom group did not score as well as the tutorial group, but this difference was not statistically significant (Mann-Whitney U = 191.5, p = .370). Clearly the two kinds of training (tutorial and classroom) were superior to no training at all (see Table 4).

DISCUSSION AND CONCLUSIONS

There are a number of limitations of this study. The three groups were not randomly assigned but instead were a convenience sample. The outcome measure was administered immediately following the educational experience in the first two groups. No follow-up was conducted nor were students followed into their practicum experiences to see how they would apply crisis theory in the real world. Over time, it is possible that the observed differences between the groups would disappear and not translate into students' performance in their field experiences. It is also possible that the no training group realized that they were acting as some kind of control for the other classes, and were not very conscientious in filling out the outcome measure.

It was a surprise that the tutorial program was slightly superior to the classroom experience. The expectation was that the classroom experience would be the most effective educational experience, and that the computer would be at a distinct disadvantage in this head-to-head comparison. In the classroom experience whenever a student would raise a

TABLE 4. Comparison of Groups on Outcome Measure

Group	Number	Mean Score	Standard Deviation
(1) Tutorial♦	24	24.33	4.70
(2) Classroom♣	19	23.10	4.60
(3) No Training	26	18.77	4.50

♦Differences between groups 1 and 2 were significant (Mann-Whitney U = 127.5, p = 000)
♣Differences between groups 2 and 3 were significant (Mann-Whitney U = 121.5, p = 004)

question about a particular slide or example, the instructor could stop and give an immediate clarification or another example to help the student understand. In the tutorial, students could only repeat sections or go back a frame in order to try to clarify any confusion. The classroom situation is a much more potentially responsive learning environment than the computer program.

In this study, the computer went up against an experienced and effective teacher. This effectiveness was reflected in the students' positive perceptions of the classroom experience (see Table 3). What would have happened if the instructor had been mediocre or inexperienced? Even a superior instructor has good and bad days and may become bored with course content or subject matter. An effective interactive tutorial will not have bad days, yet there would be changes in the professor's performance over time.

There are a number of implications that interactive tutorials raise for social work education. The tutorial is more efficient than the classroom experience. Students completing the interactive program were finished half an hour sooner than students in the classroom presentation. Students can complete the interactive, on-line tutorials at their own pace and in their own time and are not tied to a classroom presentation. Such on-line programs lend themselves to distance education courses in which students access course material asynchronistically. This is an advantage for working and part-time students who may not have flexible schedules to attend classes during the 9-5 work day.

The computer does not discriminate against users, does not respond differentially to the student's gender and race, and provides each student with a consistent, educational experience. Unfortunately this is not so with instructors in the classroom (Bulter, 1991; Schoem, Frankel, Zuniga, & Lewis, 1993). A well-designed, interactive, on-line tutorial may be less biased, more readily available, more efficient, and more effective as an educational technology, than the traditional classroom experience. These two interactive programs can be accessed on line (suicide program–http://www.ssw.umich.edu/faculty/bseabury/rube/– and crisis program–http://www.ssw.umich.edu/faculty/bseabury/) or purchased from this author in CD-ROM format as shareware for $5 dollars (send check made out to University of Michigan, School of Social Work): Brett Seabury, School of Social Work, University of Michigan, 1080 South University, Ann Arbor, MI 48108-1106.

NOTE

1. The crisis quiz has 18 questions and the suicide quiz has 25 questions. Both quizzes require students to apply concepts from the tutorial to the interactive video. For example, the crisis quiz asks students to identify the precipitating factor in Chipper's life that has pushed him into active crisis, as well as questions about current stressors and interventions that can be taken with Chipper. The suicide quiz, for example, asks students to apply the SLAP scale to Rube, to review various risk factors, and decide how suicidal he really is.

REFERENCES

Bosco, J., & Wagner, J. (1988). A comparison of the effectiveness of interactive laser disc and classroom video tape for safety instruction of General Motors workers. *Educational Technology*, 28 (June), 15-20.

Carlson, H., Bogen, I., & Pettit, J. (1989). Designing the human factor into videodiscs for human service professionals. *Educational Technology*, 29(12), 41-43.

Falk, D., Shepard, M., Campbell, J., & Maypole, D. (1992). Current and potential applications of interactive videodiscs in social work education. *Journal of Teaching in Social Work*, 6(1), 117-136.

Goldberg, G., & Middleman, R. (1987). *Interviewing skills for the human services.* Park Forest, IL: OUTP ST Software.

Haney, H., & Leibsohn, J. (1999). *Basic counseling responses: A multimedia learning system for the helping professions.* Belmont, CA: Wadsworth.

Haney, H., & Leibsohn, J. (2001). *Basic counseling responses in groups: A multimedia learning system for the helping professions*, Belmont, CA: Wadsworth.

Lambrecht, M. (1991). *Bereavement counseling: Theoretical and clinical perspectives.* New York: The AJN Company.

Lehman, C., & Lehman, H. (2000). The interactive patient: A multimedia case simulation on the web. *The CyberMed Catalyst.* Summer, 2000, e-journal.

Leiderman, M., Guzetta, C., Struminger, L., & Monnickendam, M. (Eds.). (1993). *Technology in people services: Research, theory, and applications.* Binghamton, NY: The Haworth Press, Inc.

Leiderman, M., Guzetta, C., Struminger, L., & Monnickendam, M. (Eds.). (1993). *Technology in people services: Research, theory, and applications.* Binghamton, NY: The Haworth Press, Inc.

Maple, F. (1994). The development of goal-focused interactive videodiscs to enhance student learning in interpersonal practice methods courses. In H. Resnick (Ed.), *Electronic tools for social work practice and education.* Binghamton, NY: The Haworth Press, Inc.

Maple, F., Kleinsmith, L., & Kleinsmith, C. (1991). *Goal-focused interviewing.* Iowa City, IA: Conduit Educational Software.

Maypole, D. (1991). Interactive videodiscs in social work education. *Social Work*, 36(3), 239-241.

McNeil, B. J., & Nelson, K. R. (1991). Meta-analysis of interactive video instruction: A 10 year review of achievement effects. *Journal of Computer-Based Instruction,* 18(1), 1-6.

Resnick, H. (Ed.) (1994). *Electronic tools for social work practice and education.* Binghamton, NY: The Haworth Press, Inc.

Schoem, D., Frankel, L., Zuniga, X., & Lewis, E. (1993). The meaning of multicultural teaching: An introduction. In D. Schoem, L. Frankel, X. Zuniga, & E. Lewis (Eds.), *Multicultural teaching in the university* (pp. 1-12). Westport, CT: Praeger Press.

Seabury, B. (1993). Interactive video programs: Crisis counseling and organizational assessment. In M. Leiderman, C. Guzetta, L. Struminger, & M. Monnickendam (Eds.), *Technology in people services.* New York: The Haworth Press, Inc., 301-310.

Seabury, B., & Maple, F. (1993). Using computers to teach practice skills. *Social Work* 38(4), 430-439.

Seabury, B. (2004). On-line, computer-based, interactive simulations: Bridging classroom and field. *Journal of Technology in Human Services,* 22(1), 29-48.

Sevel, J., Cummins, L., & Madrigal, C. (1999). *Student guide and workbook for social work skills demonstrated: Beginning direct practice Cd-rom.* Needham Heights, MA: Allyn & Bacon.

Linking Social Work Students
to the Wider World
via an Asynchronous Learning Network

Susan Sarnoff

SUMMARY. Many course websites and much of the literature about them address the delivery of distance education. However, course websites are also useful for bringing the world to campus-based social work students, as well as for communicating between classes and making up for missed sessions. Course websites can incorporate synchronous or asynchronous features, but the latter are far more appropriate to social work education, because students face such diverse time demands from their field internships. Asynchronous websites permit students to access posted material whenever convenient, without having to mesh their schedules with those of faculty, fellow students, or others. These websites need not be elaborate–they need only to fit the course content they will contain. However, they must be technologically sophisticated enough to prepare students to use technology in their careers; and must also reflect social work values. These include requirements that websites are accessible to students regardless of disabling conditions and eco-

Susan Sarnoff, DSW, is Assistant Professor, Ohio University, Department of Social Work, Morton Hall 416, Athens, OH 45701 (E-mail: sarnoff@ohio.edu).

[Haworth co-indexing entry note]: "Linking Social Work Students to the Wider World via an Asynchronous Learning Network." Sarnoff, Susan. Co-published simultaneously in *Journal of Teaching in Social Work* (The Haworth Social Work Practice Press, an imprint of The Haworth Press, Inc.) Vol. 25, No. 1/2, 2005, pp. 117-127; and: *Technology in Social Work Education and Curriculum: The High Tech, High Touch Social Work Educator* (ed: Richard L. Beaulaurier, and Martha Haffey) The Haworth Social Work Practice Press, an imprint of The Haworth Press, Inc., 2005, pp. 117-127. Single or multiple copies of this article are available for a fee from The Haworth Document Delivery Service [1-800-HAWORTH, 9:00 a.m. - 5:00 p.m. (EST). E-mail address: docdelivery@haworthpress.com].

nomic, geographic and other forms of marginalization, facilitating more and more extensive interactions with policymakers, experts, and peers. *[Article copies available for a fee from The Haworth Document Delivery Service: 1-800-HAWORTH. E-mail address: <docdelivery@haworthpress.com> Website: <http://www.HaworthPress.com> © 2005 by The Haworth Press, Inc. All rights reserved.]*

KEYWORDS. Asynchronous learning, social work education, course websites, classroom teaching

INTRODUCTION

Many course websites and much of the literature about them address the delivery of distance education, which is the provision of course content to students who are either at a geographical distance from campus and their instructors, or who cannot attend on-campus classes due to access or scheduling difficulties (Macy, 1999, Siegel et al., 1998). In fact, the development of such course websites, incorporating both synchronous (simultaneous) features, such as live chats, and asynchronous (non-simultaneous) features, such as discussion board postings, has made it possible for some students to complete entire degree programs on their own schedules and without ever entering a traditional classroom (Maloney, 1999). Course websites are not only used for degree programs, but are also useful for individual courses (Chizmar & Williams, 1997; Sarnoff, 1999), continuing education (Jennings et al., 1995) and staff training (Axelson, 1997). For instance, the PhD Program in Social Work at the University of Utah enables faculty from diverse locations to meet infrequently during the summer, then return home to continue their education online (Yaffe & Briar-Lawson, 1999).

Distance education and asynchronous learning offer solutions to problems that have made it impossible for some social work students or potential students to obtain education, continuing education and training: poor health, accessability problems, caregiving obligations, weather and travel obstacles, and scheduling conflicts, to identify only the most obvious (Schrum, 1998; Owston, 1997). These uses have reasonably received the bulk of attention because they make education accessible to a new pool of students. Yet bachelor's- and master's-level social work education, due to CSWE's mandates regarding fieldwork assignments and field oversight, are difficult to offer entirely online.

However, the same factors that make websites useful for distance education also offer benefits to those students who take courses in traditional campus classrooms. This paper will explore some of the ways that asynchronous web functions can enhance traditional classroom teaching in social work education, and note some of the ethical considerations that must be reflected in this, as in all, social work service delivery.

WHAT ARE ALNs?

Asynchronous learning networks (ALNs) consist of countless numbers of web pages, websites and electronic tools which enable students to learn without their being present at a particular point in time (Anderson, 1997-98). Resources in these learning networks are available to the student "on demand" rather than requiring the learner to be physically present or "logged on" at the same moment.

ALNs are sometimes confused with distance education, which uses a variety of synchronous and asynchronous media, including closed circuit and microwave television as well as cyberspace, to enable students to receive course content when they are far from a campus and an instructor (Rooney et al., 2000). In fact, distance education does not require electronic media: the "correspondence course" is a classic, if dated, example of asynchronous distance learning (Jennings et al., 1995). Distance education can also consist of exclusively synchronous communication, such as chat rooms and live broadcasts, which can be delivered simultaneously to many locations but which require that students receive or participate in them at the same time (Oullette, 2000).

Asynchronous learning refers to spanning time rather than distance, by enabling faculty and student users to post information for others to access whenever it is most convenient for them. Asynchronous communication is particularly useful to distance learning because spanning geography can result in dealing with students in different time zones (Owston, 1997). Even when they are not geographically dispersed, however, asynchronous communication can enable busy students to participate in educational programs despite heavy and unpredictable demands on their time, or obligations that do not conform with others' schedules. These characteristics are particularly appropriate to the needs of social work students, whose extensive time commitments to field agencies and clients inevitably result in frequent scheduling conflicts.

WHY USE ALNs TO ENHANCE
CLASSROOM-BASED INSTRUCTION?

Time and space can present obstacles to traditional students and instructors as well as to distance and nontraditional learners. The Internet has made it easier for students to locate material directly from government and professional websites, small think tanks and member organizations, rather than having to travel to specialized libraries that contain this content–and which often limit borrowing privileges to members or charge high fees for that right. These are not only in line with social work education, as policy and advocacy courses require timely information on recent and pending legislation, and practice and HBSE courses require access to the latest research on treatment effectiveness. They also increase access to information for clients as well as students and professional social workers.

Course websites can take these advantages a step further. They can make it easy for students to link to frequently-used websites, and enable faculty to pre-approve websites for relevance, usefulness and accuracy.

Social work students benefit from interaction with lawmakers, scholars and other experts, but scheduling such visits can be costly and time-consuming. For instance, faculty may invite guest speakers to their classes, incurring considerable travel costs, but individual speakers and students may have conflicts with any single scheduled time–conflicts which would also result from synchronous online chats. Bad weather or illness can also prevent a speaker from meeting a commitment or keep some students from attending a presentation. Faculty and students at rural, isolated schools have a particularly difficult time arranging such face-to-face contacts.

Asynchronous learning networks can be used to overcome these problems. Classes can host "virtual guests" from around the globe, who post statements and respond to comments and questions that students have previously posted. For instance, the author arranged to have an attorney specializing in professional ethics act as a consultant to a Social Welfare Law course taught both in the classroom and online. The attorney checked the website postings at his convenience and also occasionally commented on issues raised on the class discussion board that were not specifically directed to him. In another example, the author assigned a secondary text in a Social Policy course that engendered so much interesting class discussion that the text's author, who was nearly 1,000 miles away, was similarly invited to participate in the class discussion of his book. The first use was planned, the second serendipitous, but both added immensely to course learning and student interest.

The lower cost of such "virtual visits" means that many "guests" can participate with a single class–or with many classes at great distances from each other–or that students can contact experts on an individual basis via e-mail or discussion boards. In turn, students are not limited to a specific time and location for "virtual visits"–guests can be available at their convenience and students at theirs, by means of asynchronous communication mechanisms. Further, students with specialized concerns may, in this way, contact experts who might not be of interest to the entire class. Such interactions may also encourage social work students toward advocacy by demystifying access to prominent policymakers, authors and other experts.

Virtual visits are becoming easier and more frequent as authors and publishers increasingly develop websites to link authors, readers, students, faculty and experts online. For instance, Allyn and Bacon, a publisher of social work texts, is one of several publishers that has created websites for many of its most popular textbooks. The websites also offer suggested assignments, teaching notes, test banks, additional readings, practice tests, and links to other students and faculty using the same texts.

Less "expert" links are available, as well. *The New Social Worker* is an example of a journal for students that offers, among other features, an online newsletter and a discussion board where students can share their experiences with peers.

Yet another reason to incorporate ALNs into classroom teaching is that students need to use technology in most contemporary social work settings (Stone, 1999). It is therefore important that their training integrates technology with the topical content that they will deal with in their careers. Assignments can teach students how to locate useful resources online and can replicate "real world" practice problems and professional tools for responding to them.

Electronic links offer many advantages over print equivalents of the same content. For instance, data files can be made available in spreadsheets, permitting them to be more easily searched and analyzed. Information that changes frequently can be updated online more easily than can print formats; with the information provider, rather than the instructor, being responsible for updating time-sensitive content.

The potential for such online interaction is only beginning to be tapped. Imagine the effect if social work students across the country or across the world were to study a phenomenon in their own communities

(Weisenberg & Hutton, 1996)–then amass that data in a common data base to be searched, compared, and analyzed. Or imagine students pairing up for an assignment with peers in other parts of the world, sharing diverse cultural experiences and orientations (Schrum, 1998; Harasim, 1990).

But ALNs can also be used to solve more mundane problems of teaching and learning. For instance, they are means for students who miss classes to keep abreast of class discussion and submit make-up assignments. ALNs also facilitate collecting homework and other written assignments (Braught et al., 1998), particularly at the end of a term when students may be away. The author found a course website unexpectedly useful in helping students to catch up with coursework assigned during the week of September 11, 2001, when many students missed classes and some classes were cancelled altogether.

E-mail and discussion board threads can enhance classroom discussions (Chizmar & Williams, 1997). Online discussion also helps students who are shy or self-conscious about their spoken English to participate in class discussion, and may make it easier for some students to discuss sensitive or self-revelatory material. In addition, online discussion allows students to add to class discussion between classes, as ideas occur to them, and to gather facts and link files and references to their responses.

The author originally developed an ALN to support a classroom-based course which required considerable, diverse research and generated extensive, high-quality discussion. She prescreened research websites for relevant content, then used the course discussion board to bridge discussion between classes. She has since developed ALNs for most of her other courses, and developed a writing course to specifically take advantage of the posting feature, which enables students to peer critique each others' writing assignments online.

Challenges to Using ALNs

ALNs do pose challenges to all types of use: incompatible formats, translation needs, and time differences (including different school schedules, such as quarters and semesters) can thwart otherwise well-designed systems (Bull et al., 1999; McCollum, 1997). In addition, accessibility features must be incorporated into websites at the design end if students with sight, hearing, and other cognitive disabilities are to be accommodated by them–and if those websites are to comply with the

Americans With Disabilities Act (Sarnoff, 2000). The benefits are considerable: websites that effectively integrate accessability features can benefit students with disabilities, enabling them to work from home, enlarge text, convert text to speech, work at their own pace, and communicate in a barrier-free environment.

Translating traditional teaching styles to web teaching, even if it is only ancillary to classroom teaching, requires creativity and flexibility (Berge, 1999; Schrum, 1998; Wagner, 1997). Teachers who design websites need to consider which online features best translate their course content and teaching styles to web delivery.

Sufficient development time must be allowed (Schrum, 1998; Weisenberg & Hutton, 1996), especially when developing a first website or a website that is not created within a courseware platform. It is difficult to assess the time it may take to develop course components, particularly if the developer is not satisfied with early results, or must write HTML code and is not very adept at doing so. Faculty need to recognize that not every try will be successful, and experimentation time should be built into the design schedule (Kilian, 1997).

As sites are being developed, they should be pretested on several different types of equipment, opened in different browsers, and if accessibility features such as ALT=TEXT are incorporated, they should be tested, as well (Sarnoff, 2000). Websites will look different in different versions of browser software and on different size screens, and designers should understand the effects of these variations.

Once the faculty member has tested the site, it is useful to have people selected from the user pool, such as former or potential students, test the site as well. They may identify problems that the designer overlooked. For instance, navigation mechanisms that appear obvious to the designer may require clarification or even training if students are to be able to use them comfortably. The course should also be evaluated to determine student satisfaction and reactions that may not otherwise surface (Kolbo & Washington, 1999).

Students may need assistance with new technology (Anderson, 1997-98). Ideally, this should be part of the University's infrastructure, through specialized courses and printed and online instructions. Technology assistants in computer labs and libraries should also be trained to troubleshoot problems (Chizmar & Williams, 1997). This is one reason that it is helpful if the University uses a single course development tool across campus. And, until and unless most students have their own computers, it is important to ensure that a sufficient number of computers are available on campus to enable students who do not own their own computers to complete their assignments in a timely way.

Classroom-based students may bring additional challenges to the use of ALNs. For one, classroom-based students may be more reluctant than distance learners to access websites, in part because their computer skills may be less advanced, and in part because the utility of the website may be less obvious to them. Classroom-based students may also be less willing to post comments to public discussion boards, whether they respond to classmates' ideas or express their own, because they may not be comfortable facing their classmates after their comments have been posted. However, once these obstacles are overcome, students learn to be more effective independent learners when using the web as a component of their learning (Schrum, 1998).

Students may need encouragement to use the new technology (Stone, 1999). This is true whether they are novice computer users or consider themselves technophiles, because using courseware is different from web surfing, game playing, document creation, and other computer activities with which students tend to be most familiar.

One way to facilitate student use is to introduce students to the course site in the classroom. This not only permits students to become familiar with site features and navigation, but makes the website a real component of the class.

Another way to encourage participation is to require it for credit or extra credit. Yet another is to offer credit for the effort of posting rather than the quality of posts, at least at early stages (Sarnoff, 1999). Grades can be adjusted for the timeliness and frequency of posts, and only later for quality and form, as well.

Finally, it is important to keep in mind the reason that the course website is being developed. It is easy to get caught up in the trap of "technology for technology's sake," using features just because they exist, including elaborate graphics, audio effects, and video streaming because it is possible to do so (Chizmar & Williams, 1997). Even discounting the time it takes away from course content to learn these new technologies, it is vital to recognize that each new technology:

- makes it more difficult for students to access course content (because they may be unfamiliar with new technology or because new technology often has "bugs" that can only be eliminated after they have been identified by early users);

- poses additional challenges for students with special accessibility needs (because many new technologies are not designed with the needs of users with disabilities in mind);
- makes loading time and performance slower–especially for students with older hardware and software and slower internet connections.

The alternative is not to develop a "bare bones" website, devoid of any technological sophistication. Instead, it is to let course content dictate the technology used. Technology selection should be dictated by which software best accommodates course material–unless the technology is so advanced that it will not be easily accessible to most students, or by most students' computer systems (Schrum, 1998; Chizmar & Williams, 1997). For instance, video streaming technology still cannot be accessed by many older computer systems–and even updated systems may take a great deal of time to load it and play it back, especially if students rely upon dial-up connections. Such frustrations should be avoided unless the technology is absolutely vital. In this example, making conventional videotapes or CD-ROMs available to students would be a more practical option, particularly when students meet in the classroom at least occasionally.

CONCLUSION

Asynchronous learning networks serve many purposes. Among them, but often overlooked, is classroom support, enabling social work students to contact websites and interact with individuals at a distance, communicate between classes and make up missed classes; and enabling social work students with special needs to customize their learning environments. Asynchronous learning is particularly useful in social work education, because students have so many and such diverse schedule demands due to fieldwork, school work, and travel between school and field. These demands make it extremely difficult to schedule real time meetings, whether face-to-face or online, in which all students can participate without compromising field experiences. Asynchronous learning networks do not need to be elaborate–they need to be selected according to the learning needs of students, and in this way can create an enhancement to classroom learning particularly appropriate to social work education.

REFERENCES

Anderson, M. D. (1997-98). Critical elements of an Internet based synchronous distance education course *Journal of Educational Technology Systems*, 28(4), 383-388.

Axelson, M. (1997). Anytime, anywhere learning, *Distance Learning*, December 15.

Berge, Z. L. (1999). Interaction in post-secondary web-based learning, *Educational Technology*, January/February.

Braught, G. W., Laws, P. W., and Ward, D. (1998). Collecting homework on the Web, *Syllabus*, October.

Bull, G., Dawson K., Mason, C., and Bull, G. (1999). Shared communities and electronic cul de sacs. *Coalition for Innovation in Teacher Education*, Working Paper #1, January.

Chizmar, J. F., and Williams, D. B. (1997). *Internet delivery of instruction: Issues of best teaching practice, administrative hurdles, and old-fashioned politics.* Presented at CAUSE 97, Annual Conference, Orlando, FL.

Harasim, L. M. (1990). Online education: An environment for collaboration and intellectual amplification. In L. M. Harasim (Ed.), *Online education: Perspectives on a new environment.* NewYork: Praeger.

Jennings, J., Siegel E., and Conklin, J. J. (1995). Social work education and distance learning: Applications for continuing education. *Journal of Continuing Social Work Education*, 6(3).

Kilian, C. (1997). F2F: Why teach online? *Educom Review*, July/August.

Kolbo, J. R., and Washington, E. M. (1999). *Design and development of online courses.* Presented at the 3rd Annual Technology Conference for Social Work Education and Practice. Charleston, SC, September.

Macy, J. (1999). *Making the difference: Reports from distance MSW graduates regarding essential supports.* Presented at the 3rd Annual Technology Conference for Social Work Education and Practice, Charleston, SC, September.

Maloney, W. A. (1999). Brick and mortar campuses go online. *Academe*, September-October.

McCollum, K. (1997). Colleges sort through vast store of tools for designing web courses. *Chronicle of Higher Education*, October.

Oullette, P. M. (2000). *Integrating telelearning principles in web-enhanced social work practice courses.* Presented at the 4th Annual Technology Conference for Social Work Education and Practice, Charleston, SC, August.

Owston, R. D. (1997). The World Wide Web: A technology to enhance teaching and learning? *Educational Researcher*, March.

Rooney, R. H., Hollister, D., Freddolino, P., and Macy, J. *Evaluation of distance education programs in social work.* Presented at the 4th Annual Technology Conference for Social Work Education and Practice, Charleston, SC, August.

Sarnoff, S. (1999). *Development of a web-based social welfare law course.* Presented at the 3rd Annual Technology Conference for Social Work Education and Practice, Charleston, SC, September.

_____(2000). *Ensuring that websites are ADA compliant.* (2000). Presented at the 4th Annual Technology Conference for Social Work Education and Practice, Charleston, SC, August.

Schrum, L. (1998). On-line education: A study of emerging pedagogy. *Adult learning and the Internet.* San Francisco: Jossey-Bass.

Siegel, E., Jennings J. G., Conklin, J., and Napoletano Flynn, S. A. (1998). Distance learning in social work education: Results and implications of a national survey. *Journal of Social Work Education,* Vol. 34, No. 1, Winter.

Stone, G. (1999). Evaluation of an effort to improve students' attitudes toward technology. *Affilia,* Fall.

Wagner, E. D. (1997). Interactivity: From agents to outcomes. *New directions for teaching and learning,* no. 71, Fall.

Weisenberg, F., and Hutton, S. (1996). Teaching a graduate program using computer-mediated conferencing software. *Journal of Distance Education,* 11(1), 83-100.

Yaffe, J., and Briar-Lawson, K. (1999). *The distance-delivered PhD at the University of Utah.* Presented at the 3rd Annual Technology Conference for Social Work Education and Practice, Charleston, SC, September.

Responding
to CSWE Technology Guidelines:
A Literature Review and Four Approaches
to Computerization

Richard L. Beaulaurier
Matthew A. Radisch

SUMMARY. In spite of the dramatic increase in the volume of information on computer technology in social work, very little has been written about how this technology might be incorporated into existing curricula. What is needed is an overview of how computers have been used in social work practice and in educational settings that can serve as a starting point for social work faculty who are in the process of computerizing aspects classes and curricula. An extensive survey of the literature explored and classified literature on computing in social work by teaching style and curriculum content area. The authors discuss these approaches

---

Richard L. Beaulaurier, MSW, PhD, is Associate Professor, Florida International University, School of Social Work, Miami FL. Matthew A. Radisch, MSW, is a Social Worker for San Mateo County, CA (E-mail: mradisch@hotmail.com).

Address correspondence to: Richard L. Beaulaurier, PhD, Florida International University, School of Social Work, 11200 Southwest 8th Street, HLS II 364B, Miami, FL 33199 (E-mail: beau@fiu.edu).

[Haworth co-indexing entry note]: "Responding to CSWE Technology Guidelines: A Literature Review and Four Approaches to Computerization." Beaulaurier, Richard L., and Matthew A. Radisch. Co-published simultaneously in *Journal of Teaching in Social Work* (The Haworth Social Work Practice Press, an imprint of The Haworth Press, Inc.) Vol. 25, No. 1/2, 2005, pp. 129-150; and: *Technology in Social Work Education and Curriculum: The High Tech, High Touch Social Work Educator* (ed: Richard L. Beaulaurier, and Martha Haffey) The Haworth Social Work Practice Press, an imprint of The Haworth Press, Inc., 2005, pp. 129-150. Single or multiple copies of this article are available for a fee from The Haworth Document Delivery Service [1-800-HAWORTH, 9:00 a.m. - 5:00 p.m. (EST). E-mail address: docdelivery@haworthpress.com].

Available online at http://www.haworthpress.com/web/JTSW
Digital Object Identifier: 10.1300/J067v25n01_09

and consider how computer applications developed for practice settings might be adapted and incorporated into social work educational settings. *[Article copies available for a fee from The Haworth Document Delivery Service: 1-800-HAWORTH. E-mail address: <docdelivery@haworthpress.com> Website: <http://www.HaworthPress.com> © 2005 by The Haworth Press, Inc. All rights reserved.]*

KEYWORDS. Computers, CSWE, accreditation, social work education, curriculum development

Recent CSWE accreditation standards call for the integration of relevant computer technology content into bachelor and master-level social work curricula. The current guidelines allow social work programs considerable flexibility in the integration of new technologies (Commission on Accreditation, 1994). However, there are no clear standards for integration of these technologies (Beaulaurier and Taylor, 1998; Beaulaurier, in this volume).

INITIAL CONSIDERATIONS

A great deal has been written about the use of computer applications in social services. Most social work educators are probably aware of the journal *Computers in Human Services* (which has changed its name recently to the *Journal of Technology in Human Services*) that has been devoted since its inception to the development of computer hardware and software for use by social work practitioners. Moreover, journals such as *Journal of Teaching in Social Work* and the *Journal of Social Work Education* have had an increasing number of articles, special sections and editions devoted to computer technology in the social work classroom. For the past several years the University of South Carolina has held a highly successful conference on this topic. Listservs, World Wide Web sites and the easy access to e-mail by social work educators have also helped to forge opportunities for social work faculty to stay abreast of the most recent computer applications and their uses in social work practice and education.

In spite of the dramatic increase in the volume of information on computer technology in social work, very little has been written about how this technology might be incorporated into existing social work curricula. Most of the social work literature related to computing is devoted to the use of individual computer applications, with little or no explicit reference to more global considerations of how to incorporate computer technology into the curriculum. In an environment where there is already limited space for existing course content, questions about the value computers add to the curriculum as a whole have remained largely unanswered. Faculty may even be tempted to resist computerization if it is seen to take time and resources away from other substantive areas of the curriculum. What is needed is an overview of how computers have been used in social work practice and in educational settings that can serve as a starting point for programs that are in the process of computerizing aspects of their curricula.

The authors used a matrix approach suggested by Beaulaurier and Taylor (1998) in the development of this literature review. Articles were classified in the matrix based on the best fit with respect to educational style and curriculum area. To the extent possible the authors have avoided cross-listing literature in more than one cell, although this was not always possible (see Appendix). The result was a visual representation of the way computer applications might be used (or have been used) in the major curriculum areas mandated by the Council on Social Work Education (Commission on Accreditation, 1994).

The authors reviewed and classified computer applications appearing in the human services literature.[1] Each article was read and discussed by both authors until they could agree about how to categorize the citation. Relevance and applicability to curriculum followed CSWE Commission on Accreditation standards. Many articles that were relevant in some way to social work practice were rejected after an initial review as not relevant enough for *social work education*; in the end, 104 citations were classified in the matrix. Content areas included human behavior and the social environment, social welfare policy, direct social work practice, macro social work practice, research, field practicum, as well as a "miscellaneous" category that included special populations, social work values and ethics, computer literacy, and curriculum development.

Developing this matrix proved very useful to the authors in determining where particular applications fit in the social work curriculum, particularly in relation to how the various applications can or do contribute to teaching and student learning. The literature suggests that social work educators have used computer applications in at least four ways: (1) as audio-visual aids, (2) as autodidactic learning devices, (3) as topics in-and-of themselves, and as (4) ancillary materials.

The use of computer technology in distance education is also receiving increasing attention in the social work literature, especially in social work conference presentations that have an educational focus. However, issues related to distance education are complex, as are the highly specialized hardware and software packages used in this application of computer technology. The authors believed that this topic would be better addressed in a separate article devoted fully to the use of computer technology in distance education, and therefore do not address such applications in this article.

COMPUTERS USED AS AUDIO-VISUAL AIDS

Audio-visual approaches generally use the output of a single computer, projected in some way so that it is visible and audible by an entire class. The use of computers and computer applications in this way may be considerably more widespread than its discussion in the social work literature suggests. No articles were found that reviewed the use of applications commonly found in popular "office suites." Journal articles tend to focus on technologies that are highly specialized and at least close to the "cutting edge." These applications may be considered too mundane to appear frequently in journal articles, however such applications may be quite useful in teaching social work students. The authors are aware of instructors, for example, who use graphical presentation programs such as Powerpoint to do what in an earlier time they would have done with overhead projector slides. This approach to audio-visual aids has the advantage that it can incorporate sound, color, motion and professional graphics, yet can be customized easily. Spreadsheets, word processors, Web-browsers and other applications can be used similarly, and all such presentations can be saved, printed and distributed in a variety of ways. Some instructors have taken this to quite sophisticated levels using videodisk technology to create multi-media productions which combine video, audio, slide, and text presentation, that can be customized for each classroom use (Maple, 1994). One indication that instructors are using this technology is that it is beginning to appear on the World Wide Web (e.g., http://www2.uta.edu/cussn/courses/default. htm; http://www.bc.edu/bc_org/avp/gssw/sw851s.html; http://www. fiu.edu/~renzbeau/fff/fffinfo.htm).

The use of rather simple computer technology as an audio-visual aid is arguably the cheapest and easiest computer technology to add to unaltered classrooms. It requires little more than a laptop computer and portable projection device. Moreover, the examples given cut across curriculum areas. Thus, use of computers as audio-visual aids may be an attractive first step in computerizing aspects of social work curricula.

This is not to say that all software that has audio-visual applications is unsophisticated. To the contrary, in recent years there has been a virtual explosion of applications with a social work focus that have excellent graphics and sound. Although not necessarily developed for social work classrooms, these applications can often be adapted for classroom use, particularly in direct services courses. Specialized interactive videodisc, video game, multimedia, and hypertext applications can give students an interesting alternative to traditional teaching methods by using graphical displays and sound recordings to convey content (Engen et al., 1994; Maple, 1994; Olevitch and Hagan, 1994; Patterson et al., 1997; Satterwhite and Schoech, 1995; Seabury, 1993; Bosworth, 1994; Cahill, 1994; Seidner, Burling, and Marshall, 1996; Sherer, 1994; Kokish, 1994, #29). Since most of these applications will allow the instructor or other "user" to interact with the substantive content being presented, this form of audio-visual aid can be considerably more engaging for students than traditional video or slide presentations. Moreover, many of these applications are designed to allow students to use them autodidactically, and have therefore been cross-listed in the matrix (Appendix).

AUTODIDACTIC LEARNING DEVICES

Autodidactic learning devices (ALD) provide students with self-paced, self-directed learning experiences. In most cases they are designed for one student or "user" at a time and therefore require that all students who utilize the software have access to a computer. Most often ALD designs that appeared in the social work literature simulated direct practice situations where students engaged virtual clients. This approach has several advantages over traditional role-playing. For example, either the student or the instructor can interrupt the simulation when more time is needed to adequately discuss aspects or dynamics of the case, when the student has a question, or when the instructor wants to make a point. Such an approach has been applied to crisis counseling (Seabury, 1993), behavioral counseling (Engen et al., 1994) and family interventions (Maple, 1994). Similar approaches have been developed for training professionals in field settings (Leung, Cheung, and Stevenson, 1994; Patterson et al., 1997; Satterwhite and Schoech, 1995), as well as for educating clients

(Oakley, 1994; Olevitch and Hagan, 1994; Wark et al., 1991; Weisman, 1994). These approaches and programs could probably be adapted fairly easily for classroom use.

While less common than their micro-practice counterparts, a few ALDs were particularly appropriate for macro-practice courses, especially in the area of executive decision-making. Such programs place students in situations where they face dilemmas and make decisions related to providing cost-effective services. Students are required to confront real issues, in a simulated environment, related to how much service and service quality they can provide to clients given the parameters imposed by budget and regulatory restrictions (McClintock, 1990).

Several exemplars were also found which addressed course content typically found in social policy. Many used hypermedia and hypertext (Flynn, 1990; Gray, 1994; Patterson and Yaffe, 1994; Thomas, 1994), the same technology that creates the "links" on the World Wide Web. Patterson and Yaffe (1994) noted that hypermedia allows users to interact with and explore information in a non-linear, non-sequential manner, thus allowing them to learn and explore material in a way that reflects their own interests and preferred pace.

Like the practice-oriented ALDs, the policy-oriented applications create an environment where the user's actions lead to practical consequences. In general, these programs put the learner into situations where decisions they make have real-world consequences. For example, in the Poverty Game the user assumes the role of President of the United States, and is charged with the task of reducing poverty without increasing inflation. Bar graphs indicate levels of poverty, inflation, and time left in the President's term. The user is required to make policy choices, and receives feedback as to the consequences his/her actions have had on poverty and the economy (Gray, 1994).

Only one article reviewed software that seemed particularly relevant to human behavior and the social environment (HB & SE) coursework. A simulation game called Life Choices allows users to adopt roles where they are forced to confront life choice scenarios that correspond with developmental stages throughout the life span (Thomas, 1994).

One caution in the use of these approaches is that they can be quite time consuming. It is probably not as efficient to use games and simulations when compared to traditional text and lecture approaches. However, such applications may make up for this by impressing on the student a connection between actions and consequences that would be difficult to achieve using more traditional methods (Flynn, 1990, p. 205).

COMPUTER APPLICATIONS AS COURSE CONTENT

Autodidactic and audio-visual aids use computer technology to teach students about substantive social work content. In some cases, however, the computer technology *is* the content. It is becoming increasingly necessary to achieve a level of mastery with certain kinds of computer applications in order to accomplish the tasks inherent in some areas of social work. While many of the innovations in computer technology have made computers easier to use, these applications still take considerable time and effort to use. Applications reviewed in this section have in common that they are (a) relevant to one of the major social work curriculum areas, and (b) they require several weeks of classroom time to learn.

The best known of these applications are research-oriented programs. Social work researchers use a variety of computer software packages in their work, statistical and data management programs in particular. Consequently, research is one of the curriculum areas to which CSWE accreditation standards pay special attention (Commission on Accreditation, 1994, 2003). Most of the programs that are used for this purpose take considerable effort to learn, although computer technology is often considered essential to teaching in this area since it enhances the student's ability to process and manage data, and achieve meaningful results (Ezell, Nurius, and Balassone, 1991). Although there are exceptions (Forte, Healey, and Campbell, 1994), it is interesting to note that few research-related programs have been extensively discussed in the social work literature. This may in part be because "standards of the industry" such as SPSS, SAS, and BMDP have been familiar to researchers since the early days of computers. Today these programs have become more graphically oriented and easier to use. Common research texts used in master and bachelor-level social work research classes increasingly include assignments, examples and units that require the use of such software (Bloom, Fischer, and Orme, 1998; Cournoyer and Klein, 2000; Fortune and Reid, 1999; Frankfort-Nachmias and Leon-Guerrero, 2000; Healey et al., 1999; Ruben and Babbie, 1997; Schutt, 1999).

Increasingly, social work authors have begun to discuss the use of computerized applications for analyzing text as well as numerical data. Drisko (1998), for example, described the relative merits of ATLAS/ti, The Ethnograph, HyperRESEARCH, and NUD*IST for use in qualitative studies. However, like their quantitative counterparts, such programs tend to require considerable time and effort for students to learn and use them. One approach to incorporating computer technology that is easier to master in research coursework, is to utilize software that comes bundled with most modern personal computers. Johnson, Williams, and Kotarba (1991) suggest that in some cases word processing programs can also be used to do reasonably sophisticated qualitative analyses, especially when they are combined with other software to help manage the resulting word processing files, such as the Microsoft Binder program. Thus, word processing programs that are already familiar to most students may bridge the gap somewhat between applications which are themselves a substantial topic of the course and software that is more purely a supplement. Similarly, some social work authors have suggested the use of spreadsheets for simple quantitative analyses (Cournoyer and Klein, 2000). Spreadsheets have a similar advantage in that they are relatively common, and often simpler to use than sophisticated "stand alone" statistical applications. Moreover, social work graduates are more likely to encounter spreadsheets and word processors in their workplaces post-graduation, than sophisticated stand alone data analysis programs like SPSS or the Ethnograph. Educators should be aware, however, that while this software may be relatively familiar to students, the functions necessary to use it in research may not be, and may therefore still require the instructor to cover its use in class. Drawing from an earlier example, spreadsheet users may not be familiar with their capability for determining measures of central tendency, or performing tests of statistical significance.

In addition to coursework related to research, CSWE accreditation standards emphasize integration into the practice curriculum. Database programs are powerful aids to managing, synthesizing and presenting information and may be of particular interest to macro-practice-oriented social workers learning about management information systems. While these programs take considerable time and effort to set up and use, there are a substantial number of exemplars in the literature suggesting that knowledge of such systems may be quite useful to the practice community. Literature in this area examines problems and processes of creating such systems for a range of settings such as foster care-adoption (Oyserman and Benbenishty, 1997), hospitals (Kolodner, 1992), substance abuse programs (Branche et al., 1998), child welfare (Fancett and Hughes, 1996), and other social service settings (Becnel et al., 1998; Branche et al., 1998; Hile et al., 1998; Kaye et al., 1998; Krepcho et al., 1998; Thompson, Tucker, and Zold-Kilbourn, 1998).

It is common for organizations to hire consultants to develop database systems (Beaulaurier and Taylor , in this volume), and for this reason many faculty may decide that the benefits of learning about setting up and programming database systems are not worth the curriculum space they would require. Kettelhut (1991), however, suggests that it is desirable for social workers to be knowledgeable about the development of such systems since non-social workers generally do not understand the information needs of direct service practitioners.

Geographical information systems (GIS) have also recently emerged in the social work literature and may be of particular interest to instructors in the areas of community practice and social policy. These programs allow information stored in a database to be "plotted" on a map in such a way that students and others can see how social phenomena are distributed in an actual community. One such program, The Violence Information Network, has been described as a community data-base of statistics on violence, poverty, housing, morbidity, and mortality as they are distributed in a large metropolitan area. The authors indicated that the visual representation of such data had a greater impact on policymakers than the statistical information alone. Such technology holds considerable promise for making the implications of policy decisions concrete and visual. In practice, community social workers are also using GIS as a tool for highlighting and communicating community strengths and weaknesses, as well as to assist local agencies in grant- writing efforts by providing them with information on community characteristics and needs. An example of such a usage can be found at: http: //www.usc.edu/dept/CCR/nbrhd1.html

ANCILLARY MATERIALS

Many articles on computers in social work do not fit neatly into courses that are likely to show up in social work curricula. In many cases computer applications have been developed for uses in agencies to automate or streamline internal processes, train staff, or distribute information. Articles in this section are primarily helpful to social work educators in providing ancillary information or to supplement regular course content, in much the same way that "recommended" reading lists do. This section also presents literature that focuses on the curriculum as a whole and issues of computerization that may be of interest to all faculty.

A number of applications have been developed to assist in the training or continuing education of post-graduate social workers. These approaches are often quite similar to autodidactic, multimedia, and hypertext applications that have already been discussed, however the applications in this section are specialized for use by professionals in the field rather than for social work students. Vafeas (1991), for example, discusses a relatively comprehensive program that assists direct practitioners in organizing, tracking and reporting on case management activities. Other approaches help practitioners to assess, diagnose and evaluate their progress with clients (Bischoff, 1992; Nurius and Hudson, 1993; Vatterott, Callier, and Hile, 1992). A common use of computers by clinical practitioners is to streamline non-clinical aspects of their jobs, for example to construct and organize libraries of social histories (Ferriter, 1995; Zawacky et al., 1992). Indeed this is one of the earliest uses of computers by direct services professionals as noted by Clark (1988) in one of the few very early articles that still retains relevance.

There are also applications that have been appearing in the literature, particularly with regard to Web-technologies. A recent study suggests that human service practitioners use the Web to gather information on (a) service areas, (b) funding opportunities, (c) relevant laws and pending legislation, and (d) to get technical assistance and (e) to find out in what activities other organizations in their area are engaged (Stoecker and Stuber, 1997, p. 44). Moreover, electronic communication in the form of e-mail, access to databases, electronic bulletin board services, etc., can be very useful in teaching students about community organizing. Electronic data archives and communications are used by organizers to "get the word out" to a wide audience (Cordero, 1991). Such technologies are being used to help local communities stay apprised of legislative and regulatory decisions that affect their communities, as well as help them stay in closer contact with each other, and have been a tool of organizers at least through the 1990s. At a more conceptual and policy level, Imbrogno (1995) suggests that computers can be used to model social policies, in order to view the ramifications, supports and possible opposition to policies before they are implemented.

Periodically, there are reviews of websites in social work journals (Holden, Rosenberg, and Weissman, 1996) that may be helpful particularly to faculty who teach policy courses. However, many ancillary materials of interest can be found on the World Wide Web itself. There are websites devoted to keeping track of resources of interest to social workers, the best known of which is the Social Work Access Network (SWAN: http://www.sc.edu/swan/index.html). Many websites are of particular interest to policy-oriented faculty. Most policy-related organizations as well as most legislators, legislative bodies and large government agencies also have a presence on the Web. Such resources can supplement information provided in class and act as a source of up-to-the-minute information on policies in progress. Interest groups are also good sources of Internet-based information, since they often follow legislative development at their websites (see for example: www.cwla.org/cwla/publicpolicy/alerts.html; www.madnation.org/action. htm; and www.ncoa.org/). Social policy faculty may be interested in a new web resource that is devoted to state policy matters. This could be valuable as social work programs seek to meet new accreditation standards in social policy that encourage attention to the devolution of policy-making from federal to state legislative bodies (http://www. statepolicy.org/).

One caution about Web-based resources is that although they are quick and easy to access, they are not always accurate sources of information. While it is sometimes possible to get full-text versions of articles that appear in peer reviewed journals on the Web, even these are often incomplete or abridged. Most Web-based information, however, is not even subjected to journalistic standards of accuracy, let alone a peer review process.

OTHER CURRICULUM AREAS

The matrix used to classify literature that appears in the Appendix has some limitations, particularly for classifying literature on content that CSWE standards indicate should pervade the curriculum. Another problem is when the article discusses content that crosses curriculum content areas. For this reason, citations in this column of the matrix were given a code to indicate when they were related to special populations (sp), social work values (sv), computer literacy (cl), or curriculum development (cd).

Special Populations and Social Work Values

A few computer applications were identified that address the problems of special populations referred to in CSWE accreditation standards. Menon (1998) describes a fascinating example of the use of Internet chat-rooms as virtual locations that provide a safe and spontaneous forum in which people can explore personal issues that would be embarrassing or socially unacceptable in other settings. Chat rooms, by virtue of the fact that no one can directly see the user's age, gender, race, etc., make it possible to allow students to explore, and even *exchange* gender, ethnic, racial, and other identities.

Computers have also been used to help some special populations such as people with disabilities become integrated into mainstream society. The use of voice synthesizers, text enlargers, talking computers, etc., allows many people with disabilities to lead more independent lives and function in a wider variety of settings (Weber, Zimmermann, and Zink, 1995). Computers, however, can also create opportunities for discrimination. This can be overt, as when particular minorities are targeted or screened using computerized databases (Bhatti-Sinclair, 1995). Bias can also be subtle. Eastman (1991) notes that historically men have been more likely to have exposure, interest and training in computer technology than women. As knowledge of technology becomes the basis for hire and promotion, women, minorities, and poor people may be at something of a disadvantage in the work force, even in traditionally non-high technology fields such as social work. Moreover, she warns that new hierarchies may form in organizations based on knowledge of technology that disadvantage some workers by gender, race, or class. Mastery and control of computer technology by an elite has the potential to make historically disenfranchised members of society even more disempowered (Phillips, 1993). This is not merely an issue of "haves" and "have nots." As an increasing amount of data on clients (and others) is maintained in computer archives, difficulties are created for protecting client rights and their privacy (Rocheleau, 1991; Van Hove, 1995).

Computer Literacy

Articles on computer literacy tend to concentrate on what social work students should know for their professional development as social workers (Finn, 1990ab; Finn, 1995; Lamb, 1990). It is interesting to note that the applications Finn (1990a) suggested that students learn in order to become literate over a decade ago are essentially the same as the ones they would need today: word processing, spreadsheet, database and e-mail. Most of what remains for achieving computer literacy today is related to the Internet and covered in Gifford's (1998) recent article.

In general, when computer literacy has been explored explicitly in the literature, it relates to courses on computers being added to the curriculum. Finn (1990a) articulated the four criteria to guide the formulation of computer literacy courses. These included (1) the assumption of no previous computer experience or knowledge, (2) a direct relation to social work practice, (3) the promotion of mutual support among students, and (4) hands-on usage of the technologies. Finn also noted a gradual shift in student attitudes from anxiety and frustration to excitement about the power and versatility of computers. E-mail, for example, is now seen as an indispensable form of communication in agency settings, as well as between faculty and students (Finn, 1995). In contrast to social work authors who define "literacy" as facility with common software packages and operating systems that are found on most personal computers, Schwab and Wilson (1990) articulate a rather traditional view that computer literacy is incomplete without an introduction to the process of computer programming. They contend that this is necessary to ensure clear communication with software development professionals attempting to meet the needs of human services agencies. Most users today, however, will not encounter "programming" and "programming languages" except in some database applications, and it is becoming more rare even in this area. It may now be sufficient for students to have an understanding of what the various genres of software are capable of doing rather than direct knowledge of programming.

Curriculum Development

Most of the articles that have been categorized as related to curriculum development either explore the use of a particular type of computer application that can be used across the curriculum, or discuss theoretical issues that will be of interest to faculty and administrators who are implementing curriculum changes. The former include articles on the use of flexible technologies such as the World Wide Web to various aspects of the curriculum (Finn and Smith, 1997; Holden, Rosenberg, and Weissman, 1996), as well as other technologies such as computer-based testing (Sieppert and Krysik, 1996), the use of interactive video disks (Falk et al., 1992), facilitation of off-campus courses via satellite and microwave video technology (Kelley, 1993), course objectives and content in a macro-practice curriculum (Kaye, 1991), preparation and guidance for social work educators (Flynn, 1994), integrating micro and macro-practice considerations in developing information technology curricula (Monnickendam and Cnaan, 1990), and global guidelines for the use of computer technology as a learning tool (Chaiklin, 1991). These theoretical articles touch on the sort of technologies and considerations that should be factors in the computerization across social work curricula. Flynn's (1994) article is an especially good starting place for faculty interested in learning about computer uses in education that go beyond the standard office suite. Interestingly, models of computerization that have been developed by Chaiklin (1991), Hernandez and Leung (1990), and Mac-Fadden (1994) were all written before the latest CSWE Handbook on Accreditation. More recently, these computerization approaches have been updated by a model of computerization that meets current accreditation standards (Beaulaurier, 2005).

In a few cases, there are articles such as Sieppert's (1996) on computer-based testing that fell short of being models of computerization, but which are likely to be of interest to faculty in all areas of the social work curriculum. These articles have also been classified under the subcategory of "curriculum development."

CONCLUSION

CSWE accreditation standards call for the inclusion of content on technology primarily in the areas of social work practice and research. It is somewhat heartening to observe, as indicated in the Appendix, that these are precisely the areas where there has been most development in the literature. Even so, considerable work needs to be done to bring computer innovations and technologies into line with the specific objectives of courses and topic areas in the curriculum.

There has been little attention to the use of more common out-of-the-box computer technologies in the literature. Such applications may have less appeal to journal editors since they do not represent the cutting edge of current computer technology. Social work educators may want to take note that field educators–who are also employers of social work graduates–have traditionally been most interested in students having a basic understanding of computers, their operating systems and commercially available programs (Hooyman, Nurius, and Nicoll, 1990; Nurius, Hooyman, and Nicoll, 1988; Nurius, Richey, and Nicoll, 1988). It seems reasonable that emphasis should be placed on these technologies, even when they are somewhat behind the leading edge of computer development (Beaulaurier and Taylor, 1998; Finn, 1990a).

Social work educators and authors may also want to place more emphasis on Web-based technologies. Since the World Wide Web and Internet technologies have really only been well-known to the general public for about the last half-decade, it is not surprising that more has not been written about them. Still, given the rapid proliferation of such technology, it is likely that social work students will need to be increasingly well-versed in the use of Web-based technologies such as e-mail, search engines, databases, internet relay chat, browsing, telephony, video conferencing, and Web-authoring. Students will need to know about both the opportunities and the limitations of these technologies as they use and develop the potential of this technology for scientific knowledge, news distribution and gathering, grantsmanship, commerce, and so forth.

Finally, there is considerable room for empirical study of computer technology in the social work classroom and agency. Studies in this area become dated quickly, which only increases the need for up-to-date information on which technologies and pedagogical approaches are most appropriate for preparing social work students for this new millennium.

NOTE

1. From citations appearing in *Social Work Abstracts* and prominent social work textbooks.

REFERENCES

Numbers in the left margin of the References refer to the location of the citation in the matrix in the Appendix.

1. Auerbach, C., Cohen, C., Ambrose, D., Quitkin, E., and Rock, B. (1993). The design of a case management system for ALC patients: A preliminary report. *Computers in Human Services,* 9 (1/2): 33-46.
2. Auslander, G., and Cohen, M. (1995). Reliability issues in the development of computerized information systems. *Computers in Human Services,* 12 (3/4): 327-338.
3. Baker, D. R. (1991). On-line bibliometric analysis for researchers and educators. *Journal of Social Work Education,* 27 (1): 41-47.
4. Barak, D., Aloh, D., and Amara, M. (1995). Decision support system for planning and evaluating interventions in vocational rehabilitation services for the disabled. *Computers in Human Services,* 12 (3/4): 229-241.
Beaulaurier, R. L. (2005). Integrating computer content into social work curricula: A model for planning. *Journal of Teaching in Social Work.*
Beaulaurier, R. L., and Taylor, S. H. (2005). Consulting behaviors and the role of computer consultants in student learning and anxiety. *Journal of Teaching in Social Work.*
Beaulaurier, R., and Taylor, S. H. (1998). *New CSWE guidelines: Analytic tools for planning and assessing computer technology content.* Orlando, FL: Council on Social Work Education, Annual Program Meeting.
5. Becnel, J. M., Ray, S., Wolf, T. M., Lotten, T., Williams, Jr., J., Detiege, J. J., and Gable, Jr., W. (1998). The New Orleans patient tracking system (PTS): Data man-

agement for a network of community-based alcohol and drug treatment providers. *Computers in Human Services,* 14 (3/4): 73-98.

6. Benbenishty, R., and Oyserman, D. (1995). Integrated information systems for human services: A conceptual framework, methodology and technology. *Computers in Human Services,* 12 (3/4): 311-325.

7. Bhattacharyya, A. (1992). Tickler: An automated system to monitor assessment dates for psychiatric care. *Computers in Human Services,* 8 (3/4): 87-119.

Bhatti-Sinclair, K. (1995). Race equality and information technology in Europe. *Computers in Human Services,* 12 (1/2): 37-52.

8. Bischoff, R. J. (1992). A knowledge based system for assisting in differential diagnosis of chemically dependent/mentally ill patients. *Computers in Human Services,* 8 (3/4): 143-151.

9. Bloom, M., Fischer, J., and Orme, J. G. (1998). *Evaluating practice: Guidelines for the accountable professional* (3rd. ed.). Boston, MA: Allyn and Bacon.

10. Bosworth, K. (1994). Computer games and simulations as tools to reach and engage adolescents in health promotion activities. *Computers in Human Services,* 11 (1/2): 109-119.

11. Branche, R., Barron, N., Rumptz, M. H., Dempsey, E. M., and Jaeger, N. D. (1998). Management information system development for the substance abuse treatment system: The Portland target city experience. *Computers in Human Services,* 14 (3/4): 99-117.

12. Cahill, J. M. (1994). Health works: Interactive AIDS education videogames. *Computers in Human Services,* 11 (1/2): 159-176.

13. Carlson, H. L., and Falk, D. R. (1990). Interactive technology impacts on increasing cultural awareness in education for the human services. *Computers in Human Services,* 7 (3/4): 277-293.

14. Carlson, R. (1999). Using case-based reasoning to develop computerized guidance for effective practice. *Journal of Technology in Human Services,* 16 (2/3): 5-18.

15. Chaiklin, S. (1991). Using computers in community educational programs. *Computers in Human Services,* 18 (1): 73-87.

16. Clark, C. F. (1988). Computer applications in social work. *Social Work Research and Abstracts,* 24 (1): 15-19.

17. Cohen, M. E., and Auslander, G. K. (1996). Utilization of aggregate information in social work: Deductive and inductive strategies. *Computers in Human Services,* 13 (2): 17-31.

Commission on Accreditation. (1994, 2003). *Handbook of accreditation standards and procedures* (4th ed.). Alexandria, VA: Council on Social Work Education.

18. Cordero, A. (1991). Computers and community organizing: Issues and examples from New York City. *Computers in Human Services,* 8 (1): 89-103.

19. Cournoyer, D. E., and Klein, W. C. (2000). *Research methods for social work* (2nd. ed.). Boston, MA: Allyn and Bacon.

20. de Haas, L. (1995). Information technology and quality management in public social work. *Computers in Human Services,* 12 (3/4): 365-376.

21. Drisko, J. W. (1998). Using qualitative data analysis software. *Computers in Human Services,* 15 (1): 1-19.

22. Eastman, B. (1991). Women, computers, and social charity. *Computers in Human Services,* 8 (1): 41-53.

23. Engen, H. B., Finken, L. J., Luschei, N. S., and Kenney, D. (1994). Counseling simulations: An interactive videodisc approach. *Computers in Human Services,* 11 (3/4): 283-298.
24. Ezell, M., Nurius, P. S., and Balassone, M. L. (1991). Preparing computer literate social workers: An integrative approach. *Journal of Teaching in Social Work,* 5 (1): 81-99.
25. Falk, D. R., Shepard, M. F., Campbell, J. A., and Maypole, D. E. (1992). Current and potential applications of interactive videodiscs in social work education. *Journal of Teaching in Social Work,* 6 (1): 117-136.
26. Falk, D. R. (1999). The virtual community: Computer conferencing for teaching and learning social work practice. *Journal of Technology in Human Services,* 16 (2/3): 127-143.
27. Fancett, S., and Hughes, M. (1996). The development of a client record system within a non-governmental child care organization. *Computers in Human Services,* 13 (1): 63-73.
28. Ferriter, M. (1995). Automated report writing. *Computers in Human Services,* 12 (3/4): 221-228.
29. Finn, J., and Smith, M. (1997). The use of the World Wide Web by undergraduate social work education programs. *Journal of Baccalaureate Social Work,* 3 (1): 71-84.
30. Finn, J., (1996). Computer-based self-help groups: On-line recovery for addictions. *Computers in Human Services,* 13(1): 21-41.
31. Finn, J. (1990a). Experiential exercises for the development of computer literacy among social work undergraduates. *Computers in Human Services,* 7 (1/2).
    Finn, J. (1990b). Teaching computer telecommunications to social work undergraduates. *Arete,* 15 (2): 38-43.
32. Finn, J. (1995). Use of electronic mail to promote computer literacy in social work undergraduates. *Journal of Teaching in Social Work,* 12(1/2): 73-83.
33. Flynn, J. P., and MacDonald, F. (1991). Waterslides and landmines in computer-based education. *Journal of Teaching in Social Work,* 5 (1): 101-115.
34. Flynn, J. P. (1994). Practical issues for newcomers to computer-based education. *Computers in Human Services,* 11 (3/4): 359-375.
35. Flynn, J. P. (1990). Using the computer to teach and learn social policy: A report from the classroom and the field. *Computers in Human Services,* 7 (3/4): 199-209.
36. Folaron, G., and Stanley, M. (1998). Integrating library research skills into the BSW curriculum via e-mail. *Teaching in Social Work,* 17 (1/2): 3-14.
37. Forte, J. A., Healey, J., and Hunter Campbell, M. (1994). Does microcase statistical software package increase the statistical competence and comfort of undergraduate social work and social science majors? *Journal of Teaching in Social Work,* 10 (1/2): 99-115.
38. Fortune, A. E., and Reid, W. J. (1999). *Research in social work* (2nd. ed.). New York: Columbia University Press.
39. Frankfort-Nachmias, C., and Leon-Guerrero, A. (2000). *Social statistics for a diverse society* (2nd. ed.). Thousand Oaks, CA: Pine Forge Press.
40. Gifford, E. D. (1998). Social work on the internet: An introduction. *Social Work,* 43 (3): 243-250.
41. Gohagen, D. (1999). Computer-facilitated instructional strategies for education: Designing WebQuests. *Journal of Technology in Human Services,* 16 (2-3): 145-159.

42. Gray, S. H. (1994). Poverty policy software and a violent crime database as training tools. *Computers in Human Services,* 11 (3/4): 245-260.
43. Hanclova, J. (1995). Unemployment in the Czech Republic and development of an expert system for assessing unemployment compensation. *Computers in Human Services,* 12 (3/4): 257-271.
44. Healey, J. F., Boli, J., Babbie, E., and Halley, F. (1999). *Using SPSS for Windows 95.* Thousand Oaks, CA: Pine Forge Press.
45. Hernandez, S. H., and Leung, P. (1990). Implementing a social work curriculum on information technology. *Computers in Human Services,* 7 (1/2).
46. Hile, M. G., Callier, J. M., Schmoock, J., Adkins, R. E., and Cho, D. (1998). St. Louis target information system. *Computers in Human Services,* 14 (3/4): 119-137.
47. Holden, G., Rosenberg, G., and Weissman, A. (1996). World Wide Web accessible resources related to research on social work practice. *Research on Social Work Practice,* 6 (2): 236-262.
48. Hooyman, N., Nurius, P. S., and Nicoll, A. E. (1990). The perspective from the field on computer literacy training needs. *Computers in Human Services,* 7 (1/2): 95-112.
49. Howard, M. D. (1995). From oral tradition to computerization: A case study of a social work department. *Computers in Human Services,* 12 (3-4): 203-219.
50. Imbrogno, S. (1995). Teaching modeling in social welfare policy analysis. *Journal of Teaching in Social Work,* 11 (1-2): 15-30.
51. Johnson, J., Williams, M. L., and Kotarba, J. A. (1991). A microcomputer management of information system for community-based AIDS prevention ethnographic team research. *Computers in Human Services,* 8 (2): 99-118.
52. Kaye, L. W. (1991). A social work administration model curriculum in computer technology and information management. *Journal of Teaching in Social Work,* 5 (1): 49-63.
53. Kaye, R. S., Stephens, R. C., Chen, H. T., and Bruno, W. J. (1998). Development and use of information systems in the Cleveland target cities demonstration project. *Computers in Human Services,* 14 (3/4): 9-28.
Kelley, P. (1993). Teaching through telecommunications. *Journal of Teaching in Social Work,* 7 (1): 63-74.
54. Kettelhut, M. C., and Schkade, L. L. (1991). Programmers, analysts, and human service workers: Cognitive styles and task implications for system design. *Computers in Human Services,* 8 (2): 57-79.
55. Kokish, R. (1994). Experiences using a PC in play therapy with children. *Computers in Human Services,* 11 (1/2): 141-150.
56. Kolbo, J. R., and Washington, E. M. (1999). Internet-based instruction as an innovative approach to managing prerequisite curriculum content in a graduate social work program. *Journal of Technology in Human Services,* 16 (2-3): 113-125.
57. Kolodner, R. M. (1992). Mental health clinical computer applications that succeed: The VA experience. *Computers in Human Services,* 8 (3/4): 1-17.
58. Krepcho, M. A., Marks, B. J., Garnett, D. U., Snell, L., and Olson, L. (1998). Dallas target cities safety network management information system. *Computers in Human Services,* 14 (3/4): 29-49.

: 2

59. Kunkel, B. R. (1999). Technology investment trends. *Journal of Technology in Human Services*, 16 (2-3): 81-95.
60. Lamb, J. A. (1990). Teaching computer literacy to human service students. *Computers in Human Services*, 7 (1/2).
61. Lambert, M. E., Hedlund, J. L., and Vieweg, B. W. (1990). Computer simulations in mental health education: Two illustrative projects. *Computers in Human Services*, 7 (3/4): 231-245.
62. Lambert, M. E., Hedlund, J. L., and Vieweg, B. W. (1990). Computer simulations in mental health education: Current status. *Computers in Human Services*, 7 (3/4): 211-229.
63. Leung, P., Cheung, K-f. M., and Stevenson, K. M. (1994). Advancing competent social work practice: A computer-based approach to child protective service training. *Computers in Human Services*, 11 (3/4): 317-332.
64. MacFadden, R. J. (1994). IT and knowledge development in human services: Tool, paradigm, and promise. *Computers in Human Services*, 12 (3/4): 419-430.
65. Maple, F. F. (1994). The development of goal-focused interactive videodiscs to enhance student learning in interpersonal practice methods classes. *Computers in Human Services*, 11 (3/4): 333-346.
66. Margaliot, N. (1997). A model for the computerized allocation of personnel resources among local bureaus by a municipal department of social services. *Computers in Human Services*, 14 (2): 1-16.
67. McClintock, C. (1990). Caring vs. cashflow: Using computers to explore dilemmas in the human services. *Computers in Human Services*, 7 (3/4): 327-353.
Menon, G. M. (1998). Gender encounters in a virtual community: Identity formation and acceptance. *Computers in Human Services*, 15 (1): 55-69.
68. Miller, D. B., and DiGiuseppe, D. (1998). Fighting social problems with information: The development of a community database–The violence information network. *Computers in Human Services*, 15 (1): 21-34.
69. Monnickendam, M., and Cnaan, R. A. (1990). Teaching information technology to human services students: Meeting the needs of the future. *Computers in Human Services*, 7 (1/2).
Netting, F. E., Kettner, P. M., and McMurtry, S. L. (1998). *Social work macro practice* (2nd. ed.). New York: Longman.
70. Neugeboren, B. (1995). Organizational influences on management information systems in the human services. *Computers in Human Services*, 12 (3/4): 295-310.
71. Nurius, P., Hooyman, N., and Nicoll, A. E. (1988). The changing face of computer utilization in social work settings. *Journal of Social Work Education*, 24 (2): 186-197.
72. Nurius, P. S., and Hudson, W. W. (1993). *Human services: Practice, evaluation, and computers.* Pacific Grove, CA: Brooks Cole.
73. Nurius, P. S., Richey, C. A., and Nicoll, A. E. (1988). Preparation for computer usage in social work: Student consumer variables. *Journal of Social Work Education*, 24 (1): 60-68.
74. Oakley, C. (1994). SMACK: A computer driven game for at-risk teens. *Computers in Human Services*, 11 (1/2): 97-99.

75. Olevitch, B. A., and Hagan, B. J. (1994). "How to get out and stay out: The story of Cathy": An interactive videodisc simulation for psychiatric wellness education. *Computers in Human Services,* 11 (1/2): 177-188.
76. Olsen-Rando, R. A. (1994). Proposal for development of a computerized version of the talking, feeling, and doing game. *Computers in Human Services,* 11 (1/2): 69-80.
77. Ouellette, P. M. (1999). Moving toward technology-supported instruction in human service practice: The "Virtual Classroom." *Journal of Technology in Human Services,* 16 (2/3): 97-111.
78. Oyserman, D., and Benbenishty, R. (1997). Developing and implementing the integrated information system for foster care and adoption. *Computers in Human Services,* 14 (1): 1-20.
79. Patterson, D. A., and Yaffe, J. (1994). Hypermedia computer-based education in social work education. *Journal of Social Work Education,* 30 (2): 267-277.
80. Patterson, D. A., and Cloud, R. N. (1999). The application of artificial neural networks for outcome prediction in a cohort of severely mentally ill outpatients. *Journal of Technology in Human Services,* 16 (2-3): 47-61.
81. Patterson, D. A., Pullen, L, Evers, E., Champlin, D. L., and Ralson, R. (1997). An experimental evaluation of hyperCDTX: Multimedia substance abuse treatment education software. *Computers in Human Services,* 14 (1): 21-38.
82. Phillips, D. (1993). New technology and the human services: Implications for social justice. *Computers in Human Services,* 9 (3/4): 465-487.
83. Poulin, J. E., and Walter, C. A. (1990). Interviewing skills and computer assisted instruction: BSW student perceptions. *Computers in Human Services,* 7 (3/4): 179-197.
84. Rocheleau, B. (1991). Human services and the ethics of computer matching. *Computers in Human Services,* 8 (2): 37-56.
85. Ruben, A., and Babbie, E. (1997). *Research methods for social work* (3rd. ed.). Pacific Grove, CA: Brooks-Cole.
86. Satterwhite, R., and Schoech, D. (1995). Multimedia training for child protective service workers: Initial test results. *Computers in Human Services,* 12 (1/2): 81-97.
87. Schoech, D., Jensen, C., Fulks, J., and Smith, K. K. (1998). Developing and using a community databank. *Computers in Human Services,* 15 (1): 35-52.
88. Schutt, R. K. (1999). *Investigating the social world* (2nd ed.). Thousand Oaks, CA: Pine Forge Press.
89. Seabury, B. A. (1993). Interactive video programs: Crisis counseling and organizational assessment. *Computers in Human Services,* 9 (3/4): 301-310.
90. Seidner, A. L., Burling, T. A., and Marshall, G. D. (1996). Using interactive multimedia to educate high-risk patients about AIDS and sexually transmitted diseases. *Computers in Human Services,* 13 (4): 1-15.
91. Sherer, M. (1994). The effect of computerized simulation games on the moral development of youth in distress. *Computers in Human Services,* 11 (1/2): 81-95.
92. Sieppert, J. D., and Krysik, J. (1996). Computer-based testing in social work education: A preliminary exploration. *Computers in Human Services,* 13 (1): 43-61.
93. Sloan, K. A., Eldridge, K., and Evenson, R. (1992). An automated screening schedule for mental health centers. *Computers in Human Services,* 8 (3/4): 55-61.

94. Smorenburg, A. (1995). A national registration system for youth assistance. *Computers in Human Services,* 12 (3/4): 377-390.

95. Stoecker, R., and Stuber. A. C. S. (1997). Limited access: The information super-highway and Ohio's neighborhood-based organizations. *Computers in Human Services,* 14 (1): 41-57.

96. Stoelting, C., Neufeldt, A., and Hiebert, B. (1993). Development of a knowledge base for rehabilitation practitioners. *Computers in Human Services,* 9 (1/2): 137-152.

97. Thomas, D. L. (1994). Life Choices–The program and its users. *Computers in Human Services,* 11 (1/2): 189-202.

98. Thompson, R. J., Tucker, T. C., and Zold-Kilbourn, P. (1998). Development of the Detroit target cities management information system. *Computers in Human Services,* 14 (3/4): 51-71.

99. Tolman, R. M., and Edleson, J. L. (1991). Using electronic mail networks to enhance human service research collaboration. *Computers in Human Services,* 8 (2): 81-97.

100. Vafeas, J. G. (1991). Personal computer based clinical systems: A goal oriented case management model. *Computers in Human Services,* 8 (2): 21-35.

101. Van Hove, E. (1995). The legislation on privacy protection and social research. *Computers in Human Services,* 12 (1/2): 53-67.

102. Vatterott, M., Collier, J., and Hile, M. (1992). The development of the Missouri automated reinforcement assessment (MARA): An update. *Computers in Human Services,* 8 (3/4): 45-54.

103. Wark, D., Kalkman, J., Grace D., and Wales, E. (1991). An evaluation of the therapeutic learning program: Presentation with and without a computer. *Computers in Human Services,* 8 (2): 119-133.

104. Weber, H., Zimmermann, G., and Zink, K. (1995). Computer access for people with special needs. *Computers in Human Services,* 12 (1/2): 151-168.

105. Weisman, S. (1994). Computer games for the frail elderly. *Computers in Human Services,* 11 (1/2): 229-234.

106. Wier, K. R., and Robertson, J. H. (1998). Teaching geographic information systems for social work applications. *Journal of Social Work Education,* 34 (1): 81-96.

107. Zawacky, C. A., Levit, V. G., Khan, M. M., and Bhattacharyya, A. (1992). Psychiatric paperwork enhancement through quasi automated office systems development. *Computers in Human Services,* 8 (3/4): 38-85.

APPENDIX. Software Matrix: Software Type by Curriculum Area

TABLE 1. TEACHING APPROACH BY CURRICULUM AREA

	Direct Practice	Macro Practice*	Social Policy	HB&SE	Research	Other Curriculum Areas**	Field Practicum
Audio-Visual Aids	[10], [12], [23], [55], [65], [75], [81], [86], [89], [90], [91]		[79]				
Autodidactic	[23], [56], [63], [65], [74], [75], [81], [83], [86], [89], [103], [105],	[67]	[35], [42], [47], [56], [79]	[56], [97]	[56]		[56]
Computer Applications As Course Content	[80]	[2], [5], [6], [7], [11], [17], [20], [27], [43], [46], [49], [53], [54], [57], [58], [59], [66], [67], [68], [70], [78], [87], [94], [98], [96], [106]	[68], [106]		[3], [9], [19], [21], [24], [36], [37], [38], [39], [44], [51], [85], [88], [99]	[13, cd], [15, cd], [31, cl], [45, cd], [47, cd], [52, cd], [60, cl], [69, cd],	
Ancillary Materials	[1], [8], [9], [14], [16], [26], [28], [30], [41], [61], [62], [63], [72], [74], [76], [80], [83], [91], [93], [100], [102], [103], [105], [107]	[18], [95]	[35], [41], [42], [47], [50], [79]	[41], [97]	[25], [33], [101]	[4, sp], [13, cd], [22, sp], [29, cl], [32, cl], [34, cd], [40, cl] [47, cd], [64, cd], [82, sv], [84, sv], [92, cd], [101, sv], [104, sp]	[26], [48], [71], [73]

*Macro practice refers to "professionally guided intervention designed to bring about planned change in organizations and communities" (Netting, Kettner, and McMurtry, 1998, p. 6).
**In the "Other Curriculum" category, the two letters behind each citation stand for: cd–Curriculum Development; cl–Computer Literacy; sp–Special Populations; sv–Social Work Values.
(Numbers refer to References.)

PART III

Integrating Computer Content into Social Work Curricula: A Model for Planning

Richard L. Beaulaurier

SUMMARY. While recent CSWE standards focus on the need for including more relevant technological content in social work curricula, they do not offer guidance regarding how it is to be assessed and selected. Social work educators are in need of an analytic model of computerization to help them understand which technologies are most appropriate and relevant to the professional development of social work students. This article develops a flexible model that can be used by faculty to assess, develop, and evaluate computer content in their curricula. The model presents a cost-effective approach that takes into account the enormous flux and pace of change in the computer industry. *[Article copies available for a fee from The Haworth Document Delivery Service: 1-800-HAWORTH. E-mail address: <docdelivery@haworthpress.com> Website: <http://www.HaworthPress. com> © 2005 by The Haworth Press, Inc. All rights reserved.]*

KEYWORDS. Computers, CSWE, accreditation, social work education, curriculum development

Richard L. Beaulaurier, MSW, PhD, is Associate Professor, Florida International University, School of Social Work, 11200 Southwest 8th Street, HLS II 364B, Miami, FL 33199 (E-mail: beau@fiu.edu).

[Haworth co-indexing entry note]: "Integrating Computer Content into Social Work Curricula: A Model for Planning." Beaulaurier, Richard L. Co-published simultaneously in *Journal of Teaching in Social Work* (The Haworth Social Work Practice Press, an imprint of The Haworth Press, Inc.) Vol. 25, No. 1/2, 2005, pp. 153-171; and: *Technology in Social Work Education and Curriculum: The High Tech, High Touch Social Work Educator* (ed: Richard L. Beaulaurier, and Martha Haffey) The Haworth Social Work Practice Press, an imprint of The Haworth Press, Inc., 2005, pp. 153-171. Single or multiple copies of this article are available for a fee from The Haworth Document Delivery Service [1-800-HAWORTH, 9:00 a.m. - 5:00 p.m. (EST). E-mail address: docdelivery@haworthpress.com].

Digital Object Identifier: 10.1300/J067v25n01_10

INTRODUCTION

As social work moved from independent training schools to become part of major universities, pioneers such as Edith Abbott, Sophonisba Breckinridge and others advocated that professional social workers be educated in the latest scientific and practice technologies available (Wright, 1954; Costin, 1983). In keeping with this tradition, CSWE accreditation standards developed in the last decades have begun to require that master and bachelor-level social work programs include relevant content on technology. The goal is to enhance opportunities to learn about and actually utilize the latest advances in information technology for practice, research, and other curriculum areas (Commission on Accreditation, 1994, 2003). While CSWE requirements focus on the need for including more relevant technological content in practice courses, they offer neither guidance nor criteria regarding how it is to be assessed and selected. Considering the enormous variety of computer hardware, software and related technologies now available, and the rapidly accelerating rate at which manufacturers develop new and updated products, faculty and administrators can easily become overwhelmed when considering what, how and when to introduce this content to students.

CSWE's guidelines are in part a response to recent developments in the practice community which has come to be acutely aware of the need for increased levels of computerization. In recent years computer applications have been developed that are relevant to virtually every aspect of social work practice including counseling and clinical work (Bischoff, 1992; Engen et al., 1994; Kolodner, 1992; Poulin and Walter, 1990); case management (Vafeas, 1991); community practice (Cordero, 1991; Tolman and Edleson, 1991); human services administration (de Haas, 1995; Johnson, Williams, and Kotarba, 1991; Kaye, 1991; Neugeboren, 1995) and social policy (Flynn, 1990; Gray, 1994). Computer applications have even been discussed in regard to social work ethics (McClintock, 1990) and diversity (Carlson and Falk, 1990). In recent years there has been growing recognition that computers are actually changing the nature of some types of social relations, and there has been a corresponding interest in social work and related fields about computer-mediated communications, virtual communities, and cybernetically-delivered or assisted counseling and community building (Bloom and Walz, 2000; Denzendorf and Green, 2000; Falk, 1999; Finn, 1996).[1]

With the swift proliferation of new hardware and software, and the rapid rate of change that characterizes the information technologies industry it is easy to be overwhelmed by how best to incorporate such technologies into the curriculum. Social work educators are in need of an analytic model of computerization to help in understanding which technologies are (a) most appropriate for human services students, (b) necessary in order to work with clients and modern human services organizations, (c) an integrated element of practice, and (d) likely to be necessary in the future. Minimally such a model should meet CSWE standards. These requirements call for social work programs to develop innovative approaches to integrating computer and other high-technology content into their courses. Ideally, such a model should also help educators and administrators make decisions that maximize the efficient use of resources and provide students with learning experiences that will still be beneficial long after today's computers have become obsolete.

This article will develop a flexible model that can be used by faculty to assess, develop and evaluate computer content in their curricula. The model should also assist faculty in developing curricula that (1) facilitate student learning about computers, (2) create efficiencies, by eliminating redundant content and "reinventing the wheel," and (3) are cost effective. The model will also address the needs of "stakeholders" in curriculum development. Principally these include faculty, who are ultimately responsible for assessing, developing, and evaluating changes, and administrators who will oversee and fund changes. Students also have a clear stake in their learning experiences, and in many cases will be called on to make purchases, or at least acquire access to the technology being learned. Finally, knowledge of computers acquired by students should be relevant and useful to the practice community, which relies in some ways on recent graduates to inform and assist them in implementing the latest practice technologies.

A MODEL OF COMPUTERIZATION

Despite the growing importance of computers in the social work field there are few models which address how such technology fits into social work curricula, and the models that do exist were developed before the latest CSWE Handbook on Accreditation (MacFadden, 1994; Hernandez and Leung, 1990; Chaiklin, 1991). The model developed in this article seeks to update earlier work in this area as well as help faculty to meet current accreditation standards.

The proposed model is based upon four basic phases: Assessment, Planning, Implementation, and Maintenance (see Figure 1 and discussion section on each phase below).

It should be noted that this computerization model takes into account the rapid depreciation and obsolescence of computer equipment which is due to one of the four factors:

1. New technology has features or capabilities that were unavailable in earlier versions of the same technology.
2. New technology does what the old technology does, but does it easier or faster.
3. Old technology cannot be supported either because support is too expensive to be cost effective or because it is simply not available.
4. Only more recently developed technology is compatible with other new technology that has been installed elsewhere in the users' "computing environment."

FIGURE 1. Computer Planning Model

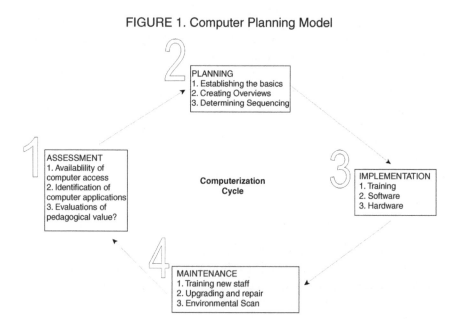

Specifically, this model will help to recognize changes in (a) the level of computerization in most social agencies and university departments and (b) the state of flux in computerization that most social agencies and university departments have undergone. The proposed model will help meet the challenge of constantly managing these changes, and the need to develop a strategy of computerization that incorporates change as a constant. Consequently, the proposed model will help administrators and other stakeholders to gain insight about goals they wish to achieve through computerization. The proposed model also stresses that these goals will almost certainly change and develop over time as new products and functions become widely available. Therefore, the model is based upon a flexible process that allows those involved to respond to changes in the computing environment that cannot be predicted in advance. At critical junctures the model also incorporates a reflective process of overview and discussion where information about current states and plans for the future are discussed with stakeholders, and where changes and course corrections can occur.

PHASES OF THE MODEL

Phase 1: Assessment

The first phase of this model assesses the need for access and use of computer technology by students and faculty. Such an approach must examine the technology that is available and evaluate the pedagogical value of incorporating these technologies into the curriculum.

Assessing Access to Computer Hardware and Software

First and foremost is the question of access. How much time and where will students be expected to use computers? How many students will need to be able to use computers at the same time? Will it be sufficient for students to use computers at home on assignments, or will they need to be able to do things with the instructor, in class?

Faculty may also want to address what students can reasonably be expected to purchase for school. Some business and law schools now require students to own a laptop computer as an entrance requirement. Social work programs may be reluctant to make such a requirement due to the financial burden that this may put on students, especially those who are already financially vulnerable or receiving financial aid. This is a reasonable concern. The price of a social work education has never been higher. Meanwhile the availability of financial aid continues to diminish. Computerization, however important, is one of the factors driving up the cost of an education (Gladieux and Swail, 1999, p. 15). These factors constitute important elements of the "digital divide" which will be discussed later in this article. Despite these barriers for some students, the price of computers continues to drop. At some point it will be reasonable to consider computers more like a textbook, which we currently ask students to buy for class, than it is like a desk, which we expect to provide.

Students also need access to the software applications they will be exposed to in class. To broaden student (and faculty) access, faculty may want to develop a policy of "sticking to the basics." Basic applications such as word processors, databases, spreadsheets, graphical presentation, statistics and the Internet are the most likely to be readily available and maintained in existing university computer facilities (Hooyman, Nurius, and Nicoll, 1990; Nurius, Hooyman, and Nicoll, 1991). These are also among the applications that most computer manufacturers today are "bundling" with new computers, with the exception of statistical packages. An emphasis on these basic applications may be particularly warranted by schools of social work in the initial phases of computerization, since this maximizes the likelihood university resources already provide some support and at least a few students and faculty will already have passing familiarity with these applications. By contrast, software and hardware that have limited or highly specialized uses are often expensive to acquire and maintain, suggesting that the pedagogical or other payoffs ought to be commensurately high, particularly when students will be expected to share the expense with purchases of their own.

Assessing the Pedagogical Value of Computer Technologies

Assessing the basic "fit" of the technology with the rest of the curriculum is another objective of the first phase of this model. The assessment includes first determining whether the computer technology provides additional benefits over non-technological approaches to faculty's work with students. Such an assessment will ascertain whether the incorporation of new technology in the classroom provides tangible benefits that go beyond traditional teaching methods.

Questions must be asked about whether the technology actually benefits and facilitates student learning in relation to course objectives and hoped-for outcomes. The experience of the author and others is that technology can actually detract from the learning of substantive course content, at times, particularly when students do not see the relevance or when they have difficulties trying to learn technologies (Latting, 1994; Finnegan and Ivanoff, 1991).

In many cases, however, computer content is essential, even if it is quite specialized and expensive. It is increasingly difficult to envision doing research, or *teaching* research (particularly at the doctoral level) without using specialized programs such as SPSS, Sysstat, or SAS for statistical analysis. Indeed, most multivariate analyses would literally be impossible without the aid of a computer. Software packages are being developed constantly for even more specialized research uses. These include programs like SingWin for analyzing single subject design data, AMOS, and LISREL for structural equation modeling, HLM5 for hierarchical linear modeling. Originally quantitative researchers were the primary beneficiaries of computer technology. Currently, however, it is becoming difficult to envision doing any but the most simple qualitative studies without the aid of software programs such as Nud*ist, NVivo, Atlas.ti, Zyquest, Ethnograph, FolioViews, and other packages.

There also appears to be a trend toward providing students at all levels with sophisticated software tools for research. Many of the more popular research texts now come packaged with data analysis software (Bloom, Fischer, and Orme, 1999; Ruben and Babbie, 2001; Schutt, 1999).

Some highly specialized software, while not important to all students, may be very important to some. This is particularly true of software that focuses directly on the academic market. Bibliographic software such as Endnote, ProCite, and Reference Manager automatically format in-text citations and reference pages at the "touch of a button." The author teaches doctoral students to use Endnote, not merely for this purpose, but also to help them organize and manage the large number of articles and books that they begin to assemble for dissertations, qualifying examinations and articles they are beginning to produce for publication. A related type of software that may become an essential research tool in the near future are the so called "Z39.50" applications. These programs use a protocol developed by the Library of Congress and the National Information Standards Organization to allow virtually all popular university research library catalogs as well as citation databases (such as OVID, Silver Platter, PsychINFO, etc.) to be read using a single program that will have the same "look and feel" no matter what database or catalog is being accessed (http://www.niso.org/ or http://www.loc.gov/z3950/agency/).

As the assessment phase comes to a close, it will be important to give faculty, administrators and other stakeholders an opportunity to discuss what has been learned. Ideally, knowledge gained in the assessment phase should generate discussion on the part of stakeholders about their interest in using new technologies, any limitations they feel there should be on computerization, their level of agreement with the assessment, and their commitment to further advances in computerization.

Phase 2: Planning

The purpose of the planning phase is to make initial determinations about how and where computer applications are placed in the curriculum. The aim is to establish (1) what the basic level of knowledge students should have, (2) how the school will provide such learning, and (3) the sequence of learning about these technologies. In this phase it will be advantageous to create overviews and graphical representations to assist faculty in working collaboratively. Faculty will need to work together to insure that those teaching advanced courses will be able to anticipate what computing knowledge they can expect students to have acquired earlier in their course of study, and to avoid duplication of efforts.

As was the case with regard to *access* to computer technology, an emphasis on the basics may increase transferability of knowledge students acquire. Social workers who have learned a program such as, for example, an early version of WordPerfect, should have little difficulty learning a more advanced or up-to-date version or a similar new program such as Microsoft Word for Office 2000. The basic word-processing functions, such as cutting and pasting, spell-checking, creating a mailing list, creating footnotes, word searching, thesaurus, etc., are remarkably similar across different brands and updates. Once a student is aware of the various functions available through word processing, this knowledge is likely to be transferable to any newer versions or different brands that the student encounters. Similarly, the same features which were basic to early spreadsheets, are still basic functions in their modern counterparts. This can also be said for other genres of software such as databases, statistical and graphic/presentation, etc. The user interface–or "look and feel"–of the programs may have been enhanced, but the basic functions have been retained. In fact, the basic genres of software applications, such as spreadsheets, word processing, database, graphical presentation, statistics, and telecommunications (Internet), have remained remarkably stable over time in regard to their basic functions and features. Examples of "early" uses of all these applications can be found in the social work literature since the 1980s when practical personal computers first began to appear on desktops (Clark, 1988; MacFadden, 1986; Gingerich, 1985).

Integrating Computer Applications into the Curriculum

The social work literature is increasingly filled with references to computer technology. However, articles in social work journals that discuss software applications rarely give clear indications about how they fit into social work curricula, even in a general way (Beaulaurier and Radisch, 2005). Moreover, faculties and administrators preparing for accreditation need an overview of how computerization has pervaded the curriculum (Commission on Accreditation, 1994, 2003).

A visual aid, such as the matrix in Figure 2, may be of some help in facilitating discussion. Figure 2 shows how administrators and faculty members might integrate computer content into a macro practice course sequence. Rows of this chart demonstrate the *breadth*, or range of courses, in the sequence. Rows in the matrix in Figure 2 might be expanded to include different courses in other sequences, or different semesters. Columns indicate different types of computer applications that might be used. Cells denote the specific activities and level of proficiency students will be expected to develop in individual courses. The matrix identifies the different types of computer applications to which students are exposed. This example also shows the name of the software that students will be exposed to. The matrix is therefore able to give considerable information about how technology is being used in the curriculum virtually at a glance.

Figure 2 also gives an indication of how students will be required to attain increasing levels of skill in the use of computer technologies. For example, Figure 2 shows how a student might be asked to do progressively more sophisticated things with computers in a first year, macro practice sequence. The matrix allows faculty members to view the proficiency that will be attained with a range of software products over time and in several courses. This can facilitate and stimulate discussion among faculty about how computers could be used in a wide variety of settings and with a wide variety of purposes, as well as with different instructors. It is also immediately evident where gaps occur, as well as where efficiencies can be created by using the same software in different courses, or building on knowledge students gain earlier in the curric-

FIGURE 2. Overview of Applications by Curriculum Area and Application Type*

	World Wide Web	Databases	Spread sheets	Statistical
Fall 1st Year Admin 1	• Virtual tour of local agencies by visiting their web pages (Netscape Navigator) • Interactive chat session with agency directors (IRC)	• Class assignment to create MIS system in (MS Access) • Use library databases to create literature review for development of a proposed social program (Library specific)	• Create budget for project (MS Excel)	• Transfer data from MIS system SPSS (MS Access, SPSS) • Generate descriptive statistics of client profile
Spring 1st Year CO 1	• Obtain raw neighborhood demographic data from census bureau (Netscape Navigator) • Obtain information re. political representation (Netscape Navigator)	• Create a database template of stakeholders for community initiative (MS Access)	• Project the cost of community initiative (MS Excel) • Create pie charts to show the change in expenditures used in target neighborhood (MS Excel)	• Summarize census with descriptive statistics (SPSS)
Field Practicum	• Design an email based network for alerting community groups about policy decisions (Eudora Pro)	• Assist agency in updating information and referral database (MS Access) • Assist agency with upgrading MIS system (MS Access)	• Develop next fiscal year United Way budget for a project in agency (MS Excel)	• Transfer data from MIS system SPSS (MS Access, SPSS) • Show significance of change on key variables comparing intake to present

*Note: Software application that might be used to perform this task is noted parenthetically as an example of programs that may be familiar to educators and is not intended as an endorsement.

ulum sequence. Moreover, faculty teaching more advanced courses can be made aware of what knowledge it is reasonable to expect students to have when they arrive in class. This allows faculty to build more advanced applications into later courses.

Discussing Gaps and Flagging Commitment to Computerization

Using the matrices may have some other advantages. Faculty might, for example, be encouraged to commit themselves to learning about and using particular devices or software *before* extensive purchases for computer hardware and software are made. Moreover, this approach allows faculty to identify where they may be deficient in areas such as practice and research courses, where CSWE seems especially interested in introducing increased use of high technology (Commission on Accreditation, 1994, pp. 102-104, 141-142, 144). In such cases the overview of curriculum can facilitate discussion about how to address or resolve these issues over the course of the next accreditation cycle under CSWE's "Avenues of Renewal" (pp. 104, 144).

Once stakeholders have had an opportunity to comment on the tentative plan, a more detailed plan for implementation must be developed which includes:

- Documenting demand for new technology on the part of faculty who will implement and use it, as well as students who will be the ultimate consumers.
- A plan and a schedule for providing training and support for new technology that is to be implemented.
- A time schedule for acquiring and installing hardware and software that is as close to the time when training and support can be made available as is practical.

Phase 3: Implementation

The implementation phase can be characterized as a "just in time" approach whereby purchases, training and use of new technologies follow in quick succession, and only where there is demonstrated demand. As soon as purchases of hardware and software begin, so does the process of obsolescence. In order for users to get the full benefit of the new equipment, they need to utilize it while it is still new. This may mean thinking differently about computer technology than other capital purchases for a unit, department or even for a social service agency. For example, it is common for administrators to have money left in some of their accounts that needs to be spent at the end of the academic year. While this makes excellent sense for capital expenditures of most kinds, as well as for consumables with a reasonable shelf life, the same cannot always be said for computer equipment.

The shelf life of computer equipment tends to be quite short. In a four-month period, say from May to September, the value of a piece of computer equipment can drop quite dramatically. Moreover, if we assume that the effective life of a computer is three years, a computer purchased in the spring and not used until the fall, has an effective life of about 2.5 years. It may be more cost-effective to make purchases of items that will not depreciate when there are budget surpluses, and buy computer technology at the time users are available to make use of them, so that the equipment does not log a great deal of shelf time.

A second problem is related to the first. When computers are purchased at the end of the budget cycle in order to use up surpluses, it is common to make purchases of computer equipment on the assumption that it is wanted and will be used. When this happens, computer equipment may sit on the shelf for far longer than the length of a summer. The author has seen cases where technology that has never been out of the box becomes obsolete before it is ever used after being purchased under the premise of assumed future demand.

It also makes sense to identify the necessary software before selecting and purchasing hardware. Virtually all software has hardware requirements. If hardware is purchased and installed much in advance of software there is increased risk that this software will not even run without the purchase of even newer hardware.

Implementation should also proceed quickly. Once plans are laid, tight timelines should be made so that the equipment arrives in the shortest possible time before training. This allows faculty to begin learning about and using new equipment before it has a chance to lose much of its value.

An often neglected part of training should focus on how to get support. There are a variety of sources of support, which include the hiring of consultants, paying for a service plan from manufacturers, software houses, and usergroups. Users need to be instructed about how they can get ongoing support, and what support they are entitled to, since this will contribute to their being able to employ the new technology as quickly as possible.

Phase 4: Maintenance

Some maintenance functions will be familiar to administrators. When computers develop hardware or software problems they will need to be repaired. When new employees are brought on, they will need to be trained, and sometimes new equipment must be integrated into existing networks and other systems.

Technical Support

There are also some maintenance functions that may not be familiar. Technical assistance is one example. It can take many weeks to explore the capabilities of even common applications such as spreadsheets and word processors and this is even more often the case with specialized educational applications such as Internet courseware. Even very experienced users are constantly bumping into areas where they need help either because they were never trained in the operation they are attempting to perform, or because they do not use the application enough to *remember* their training. It is important to recognize that this is natural and normal and that *no* amount of training can completely obviate the need for technical support.

Environmental Scans

An important maintenance-phase function is the conducting of ongoing environmental scans. There have been remarkable growth and change in the computer industry since the mid 1980s. However, most of these changes have had to do with increasing utilization by a larger number of people, ease of use, falling prices and a change in emphasis with regard to the primary activities for which personal computers are used. The growth of the Internet, and the use of computers for entertainment and communication, which is not new, but *is* newly important, have also spurred growth. So has the widespread understanding that the modern workplace requires technologically savvy employees.

The environment remains very tumultuous. Prices for entry-level hardware have dropped dramatically in recent years. At the same time hardware continues to get more complex and sophisticated. As fast as hardware improves, however, software is developed that *requires* the new and improved hardware to do tasks that worked perfectly well with older technology. Meanwhile, there is a constant stream of new applications developed for the latest hardware and software much of which simply will not run on older systems. Once there is a new "platform" (e.g., hardware configuration like the CPU chip in a computer, or a new operating system like the latest version of Windows), it is no longer cost-effective for manufacturers to develop technology for older systems. Thus a part, or the entirety, of older systems becomes obsolete.

Change in the industry has the effect of creating critical junctures that occur:

- When there is a need for major upgrades–for example, one that requires the replacement of many computers in order to run new software.
- When there has been a major technical advance such that computer technology may be used for something new or newly affordable (such as the now common use of optical character recognition technology to scan documents into text).
- When there is a major change in the way computer technology is used (such as the shift in emphasis from using computers primarily to "crunch numbers" to using them for communicating).

One of the important functions of maintenance is to identify when such junctures have been reached so that administrators and faculty can make decisions about whether it is cost-effective to continue upgrading and supporting old technology, or whether to replace older equipment with a new wave of technology.

Completing the Iterative Cycle

When a critical juncture has been identified it makes sense to call for renewed discussion with stakeholders to examine the costs and benefits of implementing new technology as contrasted with maintaining older technology. Administrators and faculty may chose to continue with older technology without making major upgrades or changes in current levels of computerization, leading to a continuation of the maintenance phase. At some critical junctures, however, faculty and administration will be made aware of the need to begin a new wave of computerization. In this case the "critical juncture" becomes, in effect, a return to the assessment phase.

ONGOING CONSIDERATIONS

This is an iterative model, based on the assumption that computer technology will continue to change over time, and that, at least to some extent, the specific nature of such changes will be unpredictable, requiring periodic assessment, discussion and careful decision-making.

An emphasis on the basics will be of some help in mitigating the uncertainties of the industry. It is unlikely, for example, that we will stop using word processors, spreadsheets or statistical programs any time soon. While much has changed, the basic features and nature of most essential computing functions were already developed more than a decade ago. The advances in these areas in recent years have generally been oriented toward making computers easier to use, more accessible to an increasing number of people, and–especially recently–cheaper.

Other applications, such as the widespread use of technologies such as web browsers, which barely existed a decade ago, are far less predictable. The one thing that seems certain is that there will be more critical junctures and new waves of computerization, and that the advent of such new technologies will remain unpredictable. There will be a need to scan for emerging trends in the industry for the foreseeable future.

The Digital Divide

One of the persistent industry trends that will increasingly confront social work educators is inequity in the distribution of information technology. The term "digital divide" was coined in the mid-1990s to describe the increasing gulf between technology "haves" and "have nots" (McClure and Bertot, 2000). While the cost of owning a computer with Internet access is less than at any time in history, people of color, families below the median income and people in rural areas are not keeping pace with others in connectivity or computer access (National Telecommunications and Information Administration, 1999; Hoffman and Novak, 1998).

While most analyses of the problem of unequal access have studied individuals and households, institutions are also clearly unequal in their access to technology. Historically, African American colleges and universities have been considered particularly at risk of falling behind the pace of other institutions of higher learning. A recent study suggests that while most historically African American universities have made great strides in acquiring the latest technology and connectivity, they still tend to lag behind other institutions (Ponder, Freeman, and Myers, 2000).

Computer laboratories are probably the most common way of providing computer access to students who do not own computers. As a faculty member in a nationally recognized Hispanic serving institution, the author has observed that in recent years there has rarely been a free seat in computer user areas around campus. Presumably, these areas are being used primarily by students who do not have access to computers at home. However, although such laboratories are extremely expensive to create, staff and maintain, it is unclear what their impact is on closing the digital divide (McClure and Bertot, 2000). Since an increasing number of students now have access to a home computer, this invites questions about whether such areas are becoming "technology ghettos": places where students who have no other options gather to use computers as opening hours and demand permit, while their more affluent classmates are able to use home systems at times that are more convenient given work, school, and family responsibilities.

While the effectiveness of laboratories and computer classrooms is not known, there is evidence that some students lag behind in their access to technology, particularly in predominantly minority serving institutions. A systematic examination of historically Black colleges and universities has indicated that only 25% of their students actually own a computer. Even among these students, scholarships or financial assistance for acquiring a computer is rare (Ponder, Freeman, and Myers, 2000). What are required are strategies that help technologically disadvantaged students to access and *own* computers that provide them with Internet access.

Educational institutions need to recognize that students increasingly need to have their own computer, and that it is legitimate and necessary to seek financial assistance to acquire one. Outside sources of funding also need to be sought for computer scholarships. Organizations such as the Gates Library Foundation, PowerUp, and others that currently subsidize computerization of public libraries and schools need to study the feasibility of providing computing and Internet connectivity resources access to individuals as well. While it is becoming inconceivable that students will attend college without using a computer, many financial aid policies still do not allow for such purchases. These policies are in great need of modernization.

CONCLUSION

Standards are a beginning in promoting computerization and technology development in the curriculum, and CSWE's accreditation standards represent progress in this area. Moreover, there are special conferences sponsored by CSWE and the University of South Carolina, as well as symposia at the CSWE Annual Program Meeting (APM) that serve to develop, encourage and apply the latest innovations in computing to human services. These efforts are an important beginning and provide forums for social work educators and scholars already interested in the topic. Unfortunately, these efforts do not reach the vast majority of social work educators who are still struggling to add meaningful computer content to their curricula.

National organizations such as the NASW and CSWE should sponsor the development of "best practice models" that involve the use of computers. In particular, the goal should be to identify and evaluate the pedagogical value of computer applications that seem particularly important or helpful in educating students about clinical practice, case management, social administration, community organizing, advocacy, human behavior and the social environment, research, social policy, and other areas of social work. However, progress in this area is likely to be slowed unless social work faculty develop methods of communicating with each other that allow them to plan and implement computerization strategies that cross individual course and sequence lines. This paper has suggested an approach designed to help faculty integrate and use technology in ways that begin to allow technology to actually pervade the curriculum in ways that facilitate maximal depth and sophistication in the skill base of our graduates.

NOTE

1. Readers interested in computer applications related to a particular area of the social work curriculum may wish to consult Beaulaurier and Radisch (2005) which reviews the literature on computers in social work and classifies articles by their relevance to the major areas of the curriculum.

REFERENCES

Beaulaurier, R. L., and Radisch, M. A. (in press). Responding to CSWE technology guidelines: A literature review and four approaches to computerization. *Journal of Teaching in Social Work.*

Bischoff, R. J. (1992). A knowledge based system for assisting in differential diagnosis of chemically dependent/mentally ill patients. *Computers in Human Services,* 8 (3/4): 143-151.

Bloom, J. W., and Walz, G. R. (Eds.) (2000). *Cybercounseling and cyberlearning.* Alexandria, VA: American Counseling Association and CAPS Inc.

Bloom, M., Fischer, J., and Orme, J. G. (1999). *Evaluating practice: Guidelines for the accountable professional.* 3rd ed. Boston, MA: Allyn and Bacon.

Carlson, H. L., and Falk, D. R. (1990). Interactive technology impacts on increasing cultural awareness in education for the human services. *Computers in Human Services,* 7 (3/4): 277-293.

Chaiklin, S. (1991). Using computers in community educational programs. *Computers in Human Services,* 18 (1): 73-87.

Clark, C. F. (1988). Computer applications in social work. *Social Work Research and Abstracts,* 24 (1): 15-19.

Commission on Accreditation (1994, 2003). *Handbook of accreditation standards and procedures.* 4th ed., 5th ed. Alexandria, VA: Council on Social Work Education.

Cordero, A. (1991). Computers and community organizing: Issues and examples from New York City. *Computers in Human Services,* 8 (1): 89-103.

Costin, L. B. (1983). Edith Abbot and the Chicago influence on social work education. *Social Service Review,* 57 (1): 94-111.

de Haas, L. (1995). Information technology and quality management in public social work. *Computers in Human Services,* 12 (3/4): 365-376.

Denzendorf, P. K., and Green, R. K. (2000). Promoting computer-mediated communications in community coalitions. *Technology in Human Services,* 17 (2/3): 217-236.

Engen, H. B., Finken, L. J., Luschei, N. S., and Kenney, D. (1994). Counseling simulations: An interactive videodisc approach. *Computers in Human Services,* 11 (3/4): 283-298.

Falk, D. R. (1999). The virtual community: Computer conferencing for teaching and learning social work practice. *Journal of Technology in Human Services,* 16 (2/3): 127-143.

Finn, J. (1996). Computer-based self-help groups: On-line recovery for addictions. *Computers in Human Services,* 13 (1): 21-41.

Finnegan, D. J., and Ivanoff, A. (1991). Effects of brief computer training on attitudes toward computer use in practice: An educational experiment. *Journal of Social Work Education,* 27 (1): 73-82.

Flynn, J. P. (1990). Using the computer to teach and learn social policy: A report from the classroom and the field. *Computers in Human Services,* 7 (3/4): 199-209.

Gingerich, W. J. (1985). Report on teaching microcomputer applications in schools of social work. *Computer Applications in Social Work and Allied Professions,* 2 (3): 13-15.

Gladieux, L. E., and Swail, W. S. (1999). The virtual university and educational opportunity: Issues of equity and access for the next generation. Washington, DC: The College Board.

Gray, S. H. (1994). Poverty policy software and a violent crime database as training tools. *Computers in Human Services,* 11 (3/4): 245-260.

Hernandez, S. H., and Leung, P. (1990). Implementing a social work curriculum on information technology. *Computers in Human Services,* 7 (1/2).

Hoffman, D. L., and Novak, T. P. (1998). *Bridging the digital divide: The impact of race on computer access and internet use.* Nashville, TN: Vanderbilt University.

Hooyman, N., Nurius, P. S., and Nicoll, A. E. (1990). The perspective from the field on computer literacy training needs. *Computers in Human Services,* 7 (1/2): 95-112.

Johnson, J., Williams, M. L., and Kotarba, J. A. (1991). A microcomputer management of information system for community-based AIDS prevention ethnographic team research. *Computers in Human Services,* 8 (2): 99-118.

Kaye, L. W. (1991). A social work administration model curriculum in computer technology and information management. *Journal of Teaching in Social Work,* 5 (1): 49-63.

Kolodner, R. M. (1992). Mental health clinical computer applications that succeed: The VA experience. *Computers in Human Services,* 8 (3/4): 1-17.

Latting, J. K. (1994). Diffusion of computer-mediated communication in a graduate class: Lessons from the class from Hell. *Computers in Human Services,* 10 (3): 21-45.

MacFadden, R. J. (1994). IT and knowledge development in human services: Tool, paradigm and promise. *Computers in Human Services,* 12 (3/4): 419-430.

MacFadden, R. J. (1986). The microcomputer millennium: Transforming the small social agency. *Social Casework,* 67 (3): 160-165.

McClintock, C. (1990). Caring vs. cashflow: Using computers to explore dilemmas in the human services. *Computers in Human Services,* 7 (3/4): 327-353.

McClure, C. R., and Bertot, J. C. (2000). *Public library internet services: Impacts on the digital divide.* Washington DC: U.S. Department of Education.

National Telecommunications and Information Administration (1999). *Falling through the net: Defining the digital divide.* Washington, DC: U. S. Department of Commerce.

Neugeboren, B. (1995). Organizational influences on management information systems in the human services. *Computers in Human Services,* 12 (3/4): 295-310.

Nurius, P. S., Hooyman, N., and Nicoll, A. E. (1991). Computers in agencies: A survey baseline and planning implications. *Journal of Social Service Research,* 14 (3/4): 141-155.

Ponder, H., Freeman, M., and Myers, S. (2000). *Historically black colleges and universities: An assessment of networking and connectivity.* Washington, DC: U. S. Department of Commerce.

Poulin, J. E., and Walter, C. A. (1990). Interviewing skills and computer assisted instruction: BSW student perceptions. *Computers in Human Services,* 7 (3/4): 179-197.

Ruben, A., and Babbie, E. (2001). *Research methods for social work.* 4th ed. Pacific Grove, CA: Brooks-Cole.

Schutt, R. K. (1999). *Investigating the social world.* Thousand Oaks, CA: Pine Forge.

Tolman, R. M., and Edleson, J. L. (1991). Using electronic mail networks to enhance human service research collaboration. *Computers in Human Services,* 8 (2): 81-97.

Vafeas, J. G. (1991). Personal computer based clinical systems: A goal oriented case management model. *Computers in Human Services,* 8 (2): 21-35.

Wright, H. (1954). Three against time: Edith and Grace Abbott and Sophonisba P. Breckinridge. *Social Service Review,* 18 (1): 41-53.

Consulting Behaviors
and the Role of Computer Consultants
in Student Learning and Anxiety

Richard L. Beaulaurier

Samuel H. Taylor

SUMMARY. As computer applications are added to social work, educators are increasingly likely to encounter computer anxiety. This form of anxiety has been well-documented in the literature, including warnings that students attracted to fields that are "people professions" such as social work may be especially prone to problems.

This qualitative study used a naturalistic approach to observe and describe the behaviors and activities of computer consultants that seemed to have an effect on student anxiety. Analysis of the results indicated that some behaviors of consultants may actually have increased student feel-

Richard L. Beaulaurier, MSW, PhD, is Associate Professor, Florida International University, School of Social Work, Miami, FL. Samuel H. Taylor, DSW, is Associate Professor, University of Southern California, School of Social Work, 1243 Alvira Street, Los Angeles, CA 90035.

Address correspondence to: Richard L. Beaulaurier, Florida International University, School of Social Work, 11200 Southwest 8th Street, HLS II 364B, Miami, FL 33199 (E-mail: beau@fiu.edu).

[Haworth co-indexing entry note]: "Consulting Behaviors and the Role of Computer Consultants in Student Learning and Anxiety." Beaulaurier, Richard L., and Samuel H. Taylor. Co-published simultaneously in *Journal of Teaching in Social Work* (The Haworth Social Work Practice Press, an imprint of The Haworth Press, Inc.) Vol. 25, No. 1/2, 2005, pp. 173-190; and: *Technology in Social Work Education and Curriculum: The High Tech, High Touch Social Work Educator* (ed: Richard L. Beaulaurier, and Martha Haffey) The Haworth Social Work Practice Press, an imprint of The Haworth Press, Inc., 2005, pp. 173-190. Single or multiple copies of this article are available for a fee from The Haworth Document Delivery Service [1-800-HAWORTH, 9:00 a.m. - 5:00 p.m. (EST). E-mail address: docdelivery@haworthpress.com].

Available online at http://www.haworthpress.com/web/JTSW
© 2005 by The Haworth Press, Inc. All rights reserved.
Digital Object Identifier: 10.1300/J067v25n01_11

ings of anxiety and uncertainty, while others appeared to be quite helpful. *[Article copies available for a fee from The Haworth Document Delivery Service: 1-800-HAWORTH. E-mail address: <docdelivery@haworthpress.com> Website: <http://www. HaworthPress.com> © 2005 by The Haworth Press, Inc. All rights reserved.]*

KEYWORDS. Computer anxiety, computer consultant, qualitative research, consulting behaviors

Social work educators wishing to incorporate computer technology into their courses are often caught on the horns of a dilemma. Some students have considerable knowledge and skill at using computers while others have little, and lack access to computers in either their homes or jobs. To compound the problem, many students are resistant or anxious about using computers. The purpose of this study was to explore and describe the behaviors of computer consultants as they helped students solve computing problems. The focus was on discovering which behaviors seemed most or least helpful in alleviating computer anxiety.

COMPUTER ANXIETY

Computer anxiety is an established phenomenon that has been well-documented in literature reviews by Cambre and Cook (1985), and Mauer (1994). It may be particularly widespread among students in social work. Finn (1990) has suggested a desire to avoid machines and technology may well be one of the reasons students choose a "people profession" like social work. While not all students are anxious about learning that relies heavily on the use of computers, unevenness in their abilities can have disastrous consequences for overall group learning and the quality of the group-dynamics in the classroom (Latting, 1994). Learning for all students is likely to be enhanced if students receive computer instruction in ways that ameliorate rather than exacerbate their fears.

Computer anxiety, which is a situational form of anxiety, is manifested in some people when they are expected to use computers in their work and learning. Feelings of inadequacy and anxiety, particularly among new users, have been discussed often in the literature (Cambre & Cook, 1985; Mauer, 1994). Although there has been little formal research in the area (Cambre & Cook, 1985; Fisher, 1986; Herkimer, 1985), most empirical studies found that computer anxiety was associated with a lack of direct experience with computers (Mauer, 1994, p. 370).

Mauer (1994) also notes that attempts to reduce this form of situational anxiety by increasing student exposure to computers have produced only mixed results. Similar attempts to change the attitudes of social work students, particularly in cases where they were somewhat resistant, have also produced mixed results (Finnegan & Ivanoff, 1991; Monnickendam & Eaglstein, 1993). Such efforts are based on the assumption that if computer use is increased, the level of anxiety will decrease. Mauer (1994), however, suggests a different hypothesis, namely that a lack of anxiety about computers may be responsible for increased levels of use and experience, rather than the reverse. For many students it may be necessary to alleviate their computer anxiety *first* in order for them to acquire more experiences in which they use computers. It has also been suggested that for students who are particularly resistant to using computers, worthless or unpleasant computer training experiences may actually contribute to greater resistance in the future (Monnickendam & Eaglstein, 1993).

This suggests that *the way* students are exposed to computers may be very important in forming the kind of positive experiences that lead to future computer use. In particular, social work educators may need to help students reduce their anxiety levels in order for them to take full advantage of opportunities to learn about and use computer technology.

At present, almost all research on computer anxiety has focused on the particular personal characteristics of computer-anxious individuals (Cambre & Cook, 1985; Mauer, 1994). As previously noted, however, the most common characteristic, lack of computer experience, turns out to be problematic since no causal connection has been established between levels of computer experience and reduced or heightened computer anxiety.

With few exceptions studies have tended to ignore various other environmental factors that might lead to computer anxiety. However, it is reasonable to posit that environmental factors such as the behavior of educators and consultants, have an effect on computer anxiety and on students' subsequent development as computer users (Rosen & Weil, 1995). If behaviors which reduce student anxiety can be identified, innovative approaches that foster students' acquisition of computer knowledge might be developed. To date, however, there have been no reports of research that explored or described factors related to the behaviors of computer instructors and consultants. Such studies are needed particularly in light of findings suggesting that students' personal characteristics are not the principal problem (Mauer, 1994, p. 374).

COMPUTER CONSULTANTS

Most universities and many schools of social work employ computer consultants to help faculty and students who encounter problems. It may in fact be tempting to turn over some aspects of training and support to consultants. Good consultants are able to intervene and help faculty, students and administrators with problems as they are happening. Unlike instructional staff, consultants are expected to be flexible and able to work with a broad range of people and problems on an "as needed" basis. This can be very efficient in that consultation concentrates knowledge resources where they are most needed for solving and remediation of problems. Moreover, reliance on consultants may be an attractive option for administrators of social work units since they are usually provided and readily available to all faculty and students in public user areas and computer support departments within their universities, at minimal or no direct expense to the unit.

Computer consultants are important to the process of computerization (Flynn, 1994; Hernandez & Leung, 1990; Visser, 1995). Faculty as well as students may well need to rely on the expertise of consultants when they have problems. Access to high-quality consultation may in fact be a necessary condition for widespread technology integration in the social work curriculum. Not all faculty are as knowledgeable about computers as they would like to be. Even those faculty who are positively inclined toward integrating computer technology into their courses may be reluctant to do so if they believe that they are "on their own" if problems arise (Visser, 1995, p. 107).

Finding a consultant with the right expertise and the ability to convey it to others, is often problematic. In part, this is because computer technology changes so quickly that it is only possible for any one person to keep up with a *part* of the developments in the industry. Any mastery that a consultant develops today will be obsolete knowledge by tomorrow. Moreover, no single consultant is likely to possess all the knowledge necessary to advise faculty and administrators on every aspect of computing. This has been put humorously in the form of a riddle:

Question: How many software consultants does it take to screw in a light bulb?

Answer: I am sorry, but that is a *hardware* question, you will need to take that problem to a hardware consultant.

Another potential problem is that computer consultants are typically chosen for their knowledge of *computers*, and not for their *user-friendliness*–or a demonstrated ability to convey what they know to others. Users rarely complain about the knowledge of their consultant, but it is very common to hear complaints when consultants do not address users' basic uncertainties and anxieties (Kreuger, 1988). Such uncomfortable feelings can only be magnified when users feel the added pressure of not being able to complete their assignments until the computer question or problem is resolved. It stands to reason that the quality of instruction and assistance that students receive from such consultants and support staff will be of critical importance in school and faculty efforts to integrate this technology into courses.

In spite of the fact that most computer users have had to interact with computer consultants at some point, surprisingly little is known about the nature of these interactions. Consultants have a difficult role to perform. They need to translate complex technical processes at which they are proficient, into simple terms that a lay person can understand. This is often complicated by computer anxiety on the part of the user. It stands to reason that some will have evolved techniques for helping anxious clients. In either case the behavioral styles of consultants have seldom been studied. The primary question that this study sought to address was, what behaviors appear most effective in alleviating users' computer anxiety?

SETTING AND APPROACH

This study utilized a naturalistic observation approach as described by Patton (1987) and Strauss (1987). Computer consultants were observed in a busy, multi-user computer area in a major university. This setting was particularly advantageous for the purpose of making observations since many interactions with a variety of consultants could be easily observed and documented without attracting attention. Moreover, it was felt that computer consultants in such areas would encounter a range of computer anxiety on the part of their clients, and therefore

might have developed a repertoire of strategies and techniques for dealing with such feelings.

The study observations were made in an effort to identify the consulting behaviors and especially those that seemed most effective in dealing
with anxious students and faculty (hereafter referred to as "clients").
The intent was to identify those techniques used by consultants that
seemed to be (1) most or (2) least helpful in reducing learners' anxiety.
As we began the process of observations, we discovered that it was also
important to note whether consultants actually resolved the specific,
tangible problems that users presented. No matter how kindly or pa-
tiently consultants behaved, their value is questionable if they do not
also effectively answer a client's questions.

CONSULTING PROCESSES

Seven consulting processes were identified and described as means
of characterizing the behavior of the consultants in their interactions
with clients. These processes, which are more fully described below,
were labeled *talking, showing, explaining, fudging, documenting, referring,* and *consulting.* They are briefly described and listed along with
outcomes in Table 1. It should be noted that some of the behaviors employed by consultants actually seemed to have outcomes quite opposite
to what was intended: they seemed to increase the learner's anxiety and
uncertainty.

Talking

Talking was the most common process used by consultants. In consultations involving *talking* the consultant would either direct the client
to do something, make a statement of fact, or direct a series of questions
toward clients. This appeared to mitigate anxiety and uncertainty in
those instances when clients seemed to have relatively good knowledge
about what they were attempting to do and only needed a prompt or an
affirmation. For example, a consultant told a client "Bring up your data
set." In this particular context her comment evoked a smile and a sense
of relief, since the client already knew what a data set was and how to
"bring it up." In another similar instance a client asked the consultant
how to get rid of a file. The consultant replied with the words: "You put
it in the trash can," referring to the small picture of a "trash can" in the
corner of the screen. Again, this answer apparently reduced the uncer-

TABLE 1. Consulting Behaviors

Behavior	Definition	Change in Anxiety
Talking	Commands or questions directed toward clients or statements of fact made by the consultant	Mixed changes depending on the knowledge level of the client
Showing	Consultant goes step-by-step through the procedure with the client.	Uncertain
Explaining	Given reasons for going through a particular task or process	Reductions in anxiety usually seemed to follow
Fudging	Misleading or giving erroneous or deceptive advice	Increases in anxiety usually seemed to follow
Documenting	Giving documentation on the process	Uncertain
Consulting	Consultant seeking advice from another consultant	Uncertain
Referring	Referring the client to another source of information	Increases in anxiety usually seemed to follow

tainty of the particular client who was familiar enough with that particular process to recognize, find, and move the file to the "trash can." However, when this same response was given to an ostensibly less-knowledgeable client with a very similar problem, this client was unable to find the "trash can," let alone conceive of moving the file to it. Signs of client frustration seemed to increase, although the consulting behavior itself was virtually identical in both transactions.

Most of the consultants during the initial stages of their interactions with clients seemed to use almost identical language and jargon. It was judged that their choice of wording seemed aimed at clients with at least an *intermediate* level of computer knowledge. It was often well beyond the level that beginners could understand, yet it was almost too simple for the expert. Consultants rarely adjusted for the level of expertise of the person they were speaking with. For example, the statement "I can't help you format an ASCII data set" will be clear to someone with a moderate degree of familiarity with mainframe statistical computing. However, a beginner with only a vague idea of what is meant by "format," "data set," and "ASCII," might well be confused by this statement. The failure of consultants to adjust their language to the level of their various clients contributed substantially to our observation that less than half of the recorded incidents of *talking* actually seemed to reduce client uncertainty or anxiety. *Talking* appeared helpful in those instances where the consultants' language and jargon matched the knowledge level of the client.

Consultants' questions often seemed anxiety-provoking. A question such as "What is the column length of your data set?," however innocently intended, seemed to produce increased levels of anxiety and uncertainty especially among those who appeared not to know what "column length" meant, nor how to assess it. Even seemingly innocuous queries were capable of producing defensive reactions. One consultant asked a client "Why do you want that [program]?" Such a question required the client, who already felt somewhat insecure in his knowledge, to justify the very appropriateness of his question. In one particular case the client displayed an episode of acute stammering before he was even able to begin to try to respond.

Showing

Showing is a process where the consultant actually shows a client how to do something by taking him or her through the process in a step-by-step manner. There were two subcategories of showing: *Hands off showing* describes situations where the consultant performed tasks *for* the client. *Hands on showing* occurred when the consultant "talked" the clients through tasks but allowed the client to perform the actual keystrokes and/or motions with the computer's mouse.

It is logical to assume that *showing* reduces uncertainty at least about whether or not an operation was possible. In showing, the client actually sees the operation, while the consultant performs it step-by-step. However, *showing* seldom seemed to reduce anxiety and may not have had much of an effect on clients' feelings about whether they, themselves could perform the computer task. Going through the steps by rote may not be sufficient to reduce anxiety, or give the user confidence that they will be able to reproduce those steps. In *showing*, consultants usually did not ask about or in any way check with clients to ascertain whether they *actually understood* what they were doing. In fact, in most cases the consultants went through the steps far too quickly for clients to be able to follow along or to read the messages or text that periodically flashed onto the monitor screen. There was little evidence that clients understood what they were doing or why. The rather minimal benefits of *showing* with regard to anxiety reductions suggest that simply knowing that a task can be done may not have actually helped clients believe that *they* were capable of performing the task. It seems reasonable to speculate that clients need to feel more of a sense of personal understanding and appreciation of the process, and an acquaintanceship with the procedures and the sequences of steps being taken by the consultants, if they are to overcome their feelings of anxiety and uncertainty.

Explaining

Explaining involved offering clients reasons for going through particular processes, or for the occurrence of a particular phenomenon. *Explaining* has been divided into two subcategories.

Task explaining has to do with giving explanations that were limited to simply explaining the mechanics of the task, process or phenomenon. *Task explaining* went beyond "showing" or "talking" by informing the user *why* certain actions were necessary, *what* those actions did and *when* to do them. In one case where a client was having difficulty running a statistical program, the consultant speculated out loud about the nature of the problem, and a possible solution. She then tried out the "solution" carefully, making sure the client understood the reason for each step. She repeated this same process with the client several times until the problem was solved. While there were similarities to the process of *showing*, as described in the preceding section, this process differs in some marked ways. As the consultant went through the process of solving the problem, considerable detail was offered about the reasons for what she was doing. In *showing,* the consultant merely went through the steps without much, if any, explanation.

Process explaining, by contrast, involved explanations that were of a more general nature and not limited to the task at hand. They seemed more directed to clients' uncertainties about *their* abilities. *Process explaining* seemed more aimed at giving clients confidence by introducing them to general approaches to problem-solving that could be used in a variety of computer situations. For example, one consultant discussed the problem-solving approach that consultants themselves use when trying to find solutions to computer problems. She *explained* that the process used by consultants is one of "trial and error," wherein they keep trying things until something works, noting that this is not so different from what clients do. This type of explanation seemed designed to build clients' confidence in their own problem-solving abilities and demystify how one might go about finding solutions. *Process explaining* went well beyond simply telling someone about the mechanics of a computer process. It was more like offering a model which clients could then use. This appeared to reduce or calm their fear and worries. For example, a consultant offered reassurance to one client by saying that she would stay with him until they were both sure that *they* had solved the problem. She repeated her problem-solving approach as they worked through several errors in the clients' statistical problem, assuring him that this was normal, and that consultants used this same method. She maintained this dialog until the client's statistical program was running properly.

One consultant who seemed particularly skilled at *explaining* seemed to be doing both *task* and *process* explaining at the same time. This consultant explained the mechanics of the task, taking pains to make sure the client understood each step (*task explaining*). At the same time he modulated the tone of his voice and the affect in his speech patterns in a manner that conveyed confidence that the client could also do the job. In this way he seemed to be using *task explaining* as a principal approach while also addressing the client's fears and anxieties through *process explaining*.

Most cases of *explaining* seemed to be successful in terms of alleviating anxiety and uncertainty. This suggests that explaining may be a particularly effective tool. However, it should be noted that explaining was observed relatively infrequently. Out of the 155 consulting transactions observed in this study, only 10 were categorized as *explaining*. Although in nine of those instances client anxiety or uncertainty seemed clearly to be reduced, it would have been helpful to observe more instances of *explaining*. This is necessary before coming to any more definitive conclusions about the effectiveness of this approach.

Fudging

Fudging refers to actions by the consultants that included any of the following: communicating misinformation, misleading the client, or performing actions with the computer which seemed either counterproductive or to serve no discernible purpose. Fudging had two subcategories which have been labeled as "Pseudo-task" and "Pseudo-process" fudging. *Pseudo-task fudging* occurred when the consultant appeared to be working knowledgeably on the task at hand, but was either misleading the client, or was not able to successfully complete the problem-solving task. For example, when asked a question about how to download a computer program available from the university, one consultant went into a flurry of keyboard activity which produced no discernible result, and which appeared to the observer as the same, unsuccessful, action repeated over and over. This is characteristic of *pseudo-task fudging*; the consultant works "diligently" at a task that appears to be addressing the client's problem, but is in fact something else. In this case, an activity that looked as though it were highly technical, actually may have been stalling for time or guessing. The client may not even be aware that the consultant is fudging, but only that the problem is not being solved. In some cases this may even compound anxiety, if watching clients conclude that the task is so difficult that even the consultant, with all his/her furious and mysterious activity, seems unable to generate a solution to their problem.

Another kind of *pseudo-task fudging* occurred when consultants seemed to become so involved with technical tangents of the client's problem that they lost track of the actual question the client had asked. One client, for instance, presented a problem involving uploading files from a PC to one of the mainframe computers. The client could get the file to appear in the mainframe account, but although he could see it, he was not able to access it. The client wanted to know how to upload the files in such a way that they could be used. The consultant, however, seemed to become fascinated with the file itself and set about trying to work with and fix its problems. The client repeatedly informed the consultant that he was not interested in how to *fix* the file. What he was interested in was how to *upload the file* in such a way that it would not *need to be fixed*. The consultant was, in this case, *pseudo-task fudging* because, although she was focused on an interesting technical *aspect* of the problem, she was not working on the *client's* problem and may not have even understood how to help the client.

Like *process explaining, pseudo-process fudging* seemed on the face of it, to address either clients' anxieties or general problem-solving processes. In the case of *pseudo-process fudging*, however, the consultant was actually misleading clients or giving them a false sense of security. For example, one client sought help in downloading library information from one of the university mainframe computers. The client asked whether he would be able to download this information from the mainframe to one of the Macintosh PCs. The consultant informed him that indeed he certainly would be able to do so. In fact, however, the computers the client was using were not equipped with the necessary software to download library information. Since the consultant was misinforming the client about a basic computer task, he was engaging in *pseudo-task fudging*. However, when the client expressed worry about not knowing how to download the information, the consultant replied by saying "Don't worry, I'll be here [for the next hour]." The comment was apparently designed to address the client's anxiety. However, since this incident resulted in a total loss of the library information, the client's worries were reinforced or exacerbated.

A different type of *pseudo-process fudging* occurred when a consultant would give misinformation that seemed designed to get the client to give up on what would otherwise be a productive activity. In one case of this type of *fudging* a client asked about the availability of a particular operating system tutorial. The consultant informed the client that no such program existed. The implication was rather clear: the client should abandon the search for the program. In fact, however, the program about which the client was inquiring was available on some of the PCs in the user area.

It was quite surprising to find that *fudging* was one of the more prevalent consulting behaviors that were observed. Nearly one-quarter of all of the recorded consulting processes involved one or another type of *fudging*. This is unfortunate since it almost always seemed to provoke or stimulate heightened levels of anxiety or uncertainty. Moreover, clients exited the consultation transaction with incorrect or misleading information.

Documenting and Consulting

Three consulting activities, *documenting*, *consulting,* and *referring* seemed to have little effect on anxiety or may have actually exacerbated it. However, they were not observed very frequently. However, each of these behaviors was observed at least a few times, and may be of interest to authors thinking of conducting research in this area.

Documenting occurred when the consultant used and/or gave out handouts, manuals or other documentation prepared by the computer services department in order to answer a question. *Consulting* refers to the consultant seeking consultation with another consultant. Neither *documenting* nor *consulting* seemed to have much of an effect on clients' anxiety and uncertainty.

Referring

Referring occurred in two forms: (a) a referral to another source (i.e., another consultant or the manufacturer); or, (b) to a later point in time. Most often the consultant would refer the client to another consultant or would promise to have an answer for the client at a later time. Most often *referring* seemed to promote client anxiety and uncertainty. This may be because *referrals* were usually given at a point and in a manner by which it was unclear as to which consultants were responsible for answering clients' questions. This is a common experience for users of telephone support lines who, after waiting on the telephone for what seems to be forever, are told that they have called the wrong support line. A common example we observed involved using a PC to access a mainframe computer. It sometimes appeared that the consultant was not sure whether the question was more appropriate for mainframe or PC consultants. It seems reasonable to speculate that for some clients learning that even the computer "expert" is not able to help may be quite anxiety provoking. Further, if the consultant seems unsure about where to refer the client, that might compound client uncertainty.

It is, of course, quite possible that *documenting, consulting* and *referring* may be effective in reducing anxiety and uncertainty in ways we were not in a position to note. These behaviors were not frequently observed in this study. It seems reasonable to speculate that such activities by consultants might reduce anxiety or uncertainty in the long run, even if they did not seem to have much of a positive effect on clients in the user room. Consultations with and referrals to people outside the user area could not be observed. Future studies of the effectiveness of handouts, other types of documentation, and referrals to outside consultants need to be conducted.

DISCUSSION

The methods used and the population observed in this study do not allow for broad generalizability. Even so, it is unsettling to note that nearly 40% of the consulting processes observed in this study seemed to have exacerbated or provoked client anxiety and/or confusion. Only one-third of these consulting transactions clearly appeared to reduce client anxiety. This suggests that it may not be feasible for social work educators to assume that computer consultants will have developed appropriate and effective techniques that help students deal with their fears about using computers.

Processes such as *talking, explaining, showing, documenting, consulting,* and *referring* all appeared to have somewhat questionable or indeterminate effects. *Explaining* seemed to have the clearest potential for alleviating both anxieties and uncertainties, as does *talking*. Future researchers may be interested in whether *explaining* behaviors when combined with *showing,* can overcome some of the limitations observed when *showing* was used alone. *Showing*, all by itself, appeared to have surprisingly little effect on anxiety.

Documenting, *referring*, and *consulting* seemed to have had almost no influence on reducing clients' anxiety and uncertainty. These activities may be necessary in some situations (after all, no consultant can be expected to know everything!) but it is important that both consultants and educators remain aware of the limitations inherent in these approaches. Since this study was not able to assess the longer-term effects of consulting behaviors, future researchers also may want to examine which behaviors are helpful over time. It is quite possible that some of these observed behaviors actually helped clients but this research did not allow for this to be documented.

The most consistently destructive process observed was *fudging*. Such behaviors are probably used to mask a lack of appropriate knowledge or to allow additional time for the consultant to come up with an actual solution to client problems. A full understanding of these behaviors will require further research. In any case, consultants should probably be made aware of the potential dangers inherent in their use of *fudging*.

Using Computer Consultants

There is mounting pressure to add computer content to social work curricula. The workplace that social work students will enter increasingly features a variety of computerized information systems, electronic record keeping, telecommunications, as well as the (by now) routine word processing and spreadsheet applications. Students need to have a basic understanding of the utilization of these technologies in order to be able to function effectively. This is reflected in CSWE requirements for master and bachelor programs in social work that require students to be exposed to new technologies during their professional education (Commission on Accreditation, 1994, 2003).

There is a burgeoning agreement that what most social workers need is a level of basic "computer literacy" (Ezell, Nurius, & Balassone, 1991; Finn, 1995; Flynn, 1994; Reinoehl & Mueller, 1990). For most social work students, as well as for most faculty, an understanding of how to use basic operating systems and programs on processors, spreadsheets, databases, telecommunications, and statistical programs will suffice. Most social workers do not need the level of technical competence necessary to create specialized software applications, although some social workers can and do have these competencies.

Many social work educators see "user rooms" and computer consultants as at least a partial solution to the problem of increasing students' access to and knowledge of basic computing. There is inherent efficiency in the approach. Those students who do need help are able to receive technical assistance that applies the specific problems they are having. Those students who do not need help are not forced to sit through exercises and classroom experiences they do not need or want. The use of computer consultants to help students who are having problems with basic computing skills also has the advantage of freeing social work educators from the burdens of remedial instruction of students regarding computer basics. For example, the instructor can announce that students will need to be proficient in using such applications as an Excel spreadsheet or the Netscape Navigator web browser. Students who need help or instruction in how to use these applications should report to a computer laboratory at a specified time where consultants will be available to help them. This may allow faculty to concentrate on how specific computer technologies relate to their course material rather than forcing them to spend all-too-limited class time on the rudiments of computer use.

However, the findings raise some cautions about turning social work students over to computer consultants. Social work educators inclined to rely on the use of computer consultants may wish to screen these consultants for their "people skills." Since social workers may actually be somewhat less computer literate than their counterparts in other disciplines (Finn, 1990; Lamb, 1990), it may be necessary to do some special preparation and training with consultants to make sure they are aware of those behaviors which are particularly helpful in instructing social work students and which have the potential to exacerbate their fears and anxieties. When possible, social work educators may be inclined to consider whether consultants are really necessary, or whether there are students, doctoral students or others who already have good "people skills" who might be recruited or trained to fill positions as consultants.

In many cases, however, the use of such consultants is likely to be unavoidable, since the expertise that they bring may not be available from other sources. While this study raises several serious questions about the efficiency of some interactions with computer consultants, it is important to note that such support personnel have a vital role to play as social work units increasingly computerize parts of their curriculum (Flynn, 1994; Hernandez & Leung, 1990; Visser, 1995). This becomes even more important at a time when many software and hardware manufacturers cut back on their offers of free and available technical assistance and documentation. At one time it was common for most software packages to come with telephone book-sized manuals and toll-free telephone numbers for technical support; such "free" assistance is less usual these days. Social work programs increasingly need to rely on "in-house" sources of support. In selecting in-house consultants, however, it is important to remember what early Apple Computer commercials so effectively pointed out: that what makes computer technology efficient and effective is not so much its cost or sophistication, but whether it *actually gets used*. This adage is probably even more applicable to the role of computer consultants. The consultant will have to be able to actually come up with and communicate solutions to computer problems as presented by social workers. Just as important, however, effective consultants have to competently deal with fears and anxieties that many users continue to have in order for their technical expertise to be put to good use.

CONCLUSION AND RECOMMENDATIONS

Further research using more focused and rigorous descriptive and explanatory methods will, of course, be necessary to determine the effects that various behaviors have on computer anxiety. This study was designed as an initial exploration and effort at categorization of consultant behaviors. It would be beyond the purview of this study to suggest that these behaviors are widespread or even to speculate on how intense an effect they may have on anxiety.

Even so, the findings suggest that interpersonal skills may be very important in exchanges between consultants and computer users. This is important for a variety of reasons. First, this supports the notion that *how* students are exposed to computers is important in terms of reducing their anxieties. If Mauer (1994) is correct in suggesting that positive attitudes affect the degree to which students use computers, then this study's suggestion that there may be a direct link between learners' positive and negative attitudes about computers and the quality of instruction they receive, is especially critical. If subsequent researchers, for example, find that behaviors such as *fudging* exacerbate negative attitudes, it may well be that such instructional encounters actually tend to raise anxiety levels and even drive students away from future computer use.

This initial, exploratory study also raises the interesting notion that the effectiveness of such encounters could be enhanced if consultants received some rudimentary training in fundamental *social work* skills such as critical listening and interviewing. It seems reasonable to expect that social work educators might help prepare consultants to *start where their clients are*, by sensitizing them to the anxiety levels and knowledge gaps that may characterize many of the social work students they are likely to work with.

While this study was primarily concerned with consultants, subsequent researchers may want to investigate whether the behaviors encountered in consulting situations also appear in more mainstream computer training and learning environments. If so, educators may wish to reexamine their communication approaches and styles when teaching about the use of computers.

This study also has implications for subsequent research on computer anxiety. The findings of this study suggest that external factors such as the behavior of computer consultants very likely influence the anxiety levels of users. More rigorous descriptive and experimental designs utilizing the consultant behaviors identified in this study, may yield more knowledge as to which behaviors are ultimately most and/or least effective for reducing students' computer anxiety.

REFERENCES

Cambre, M. A., & Cook, D. L. (1985). Computer anxiety: Definition, measurement, and correlates. *Journal of Educational Computing Research, 1*(1).

Commission on Accreditation (1994, 2003). *Handbook of accreditation standards and procedures* (4th ed., 5th ed.). Alexandria, VA: Council on Social Work Education.

Ezell, M., Nurius, P. S., & Balassone, M. L. (1991). Preparing computer literate social workers: An integrative approach. *Journal of Teaching in Social Work, 5*(1), 81-99.

Finn, J. (1990). Teaching computer telecommunications to social work undergraduates. *Arete, 15*(2), 38-43.

Finn, J. (1995). Use of electronic mail to promote computer literacy in social work undergraduates. *Journal of Teaching in Social Work, 12*(1/2), 73-83.

Finnegan, D. J., & Ivanoff, A. (1991). Effects of brief computer training on attitudes toward computer use in practice: An educational experiment. *Journal of Social Work Education, 27*(1), 73-82.

Fisher, F. (1986). *Computer anxiety in special and regular education credential candidates.* Unpublished Doctoral Dissertation, University of Southern California, Los Angeles, CA.

Flynn, J. P. (1994). Practical issues for newcomers to computer-based education. *Computers in Human Services, 11*(3/4), 359-375.

Herkimer, B. (1985). *Computer anxiety as state anxiety and time-on-task and their relationship to sex, age, previous experience, and typing ability.* Unpublished Doctoral Dissertation, University of Southern California, Los Angeles, CA.

Hernandez, S. H., & Leung, P. (1990). Implementing a social work curriculum on information technology. *Computers in Human Services, 7*(1/2).

Kreuger, L. (1988). Encountering microcomputers: A phenomenological analysis. *Computers in Human Services, 3*(3-4), 71-86.

Lamb, J. A. (1990). Teaching computer literacy to human service students. *Computers in Human Services, 7*(1/2).

Latting, J. K. (1994). Diffusion of computer-mediated communication in a graduate class: Lessons from the class from Hell. *Computers in Human Services, 10*(3), 21-45.

Mauer, M. M. (1994). Computer anxiety correlates and what they tell us: A literature review. *Computers in Human Behavior, 10*(3), 369-376.

Monnickendam, M., & Eaglstein, A. S. (1993). Computer acceptance by social workers: Some unexpected research findings. *Computers in Human Services, 9*(3-4), 409-424.

Patton, M. Q. (1987). *How to use qualitative methods in evaluation.* Newbury Park, CA: Sage.

Reinoehl, R. L., & Mueller, B. J. (1990). Introducing computer literacy in human services education. *Computers in Human Services, 7*(1/2), 3-18.

Rosen, L. D., & Weil, M. M. (1995). Computer availability, computer experience and technophobia among public school teachers. *Computers in Human Behavior, 11*(1), 9-31.

Strauss, A. L. (1987). *Qualitative analysis for social scientists.* Cambridge: Cambridge University Press.

Visser, A. (1995). Computers in education: Added value leading towards better quality. *Computers in Human Services, 12*(1/2), 81-97.

The Diffusion of Information Technology in the Human Services: Implications for Social Work Education

Dale Fitch

SUMMARY. The spread and utilization of information technology in the human services is examined using innovation diffusion theory. This examination is contextualized within the values basis of social work. Literature from the human services, the business sector, and the social sciences regarding the role of information technology is used to promote a broader perspective on the issues faced in innovation diffusion in our profession. The paper concludes with implications for social work education and suggestions for future research. *[Article copies available for a fee from The Haworth Document Delivery Service: 1-800-HAWORTH. E-mail address: <docdelivery@haworthpress.com> Website: <http://www.HaworthPress.com> © 2005 by The Haworth Press, Inc. All rights reserved.]*

KEYWORDS. Information technology, social work education, innovation diffusion theory

---

Dale Fitch, PhD, is affiliated with the School of Social Work, University of Michigan, 1080 South University, Room 2794, Ann Arbor, MI 48109-1106 (E-mail: dale@umich.edu).

[Haworth co-indexing entry note]: "The Diffusion of Information Technology in the Human Services: Implications for Social Work Education." Fitch, Dale. Co-published simultaneously in *Journal of Teaching in Social Work* (The Haworth Social Work Practice Press, an imprint of The Haworth Press, Inc.) Vol. 25, No. 1/2, 2005, pp. 191-204; and: *Technology in Social Work Education and Curriculum: The High Tech, High Touch Social Work Educator* (ed: Richard L. Beaulaurier, and Martha Haffey) The Haworth Social Work Practice Press, an imprint of The Haworth Press, Inc., 2005, pp. 191-204. Single or multiple copies of this article are available for a fee from The Haworth Document Delivery Service [1-800-HAWORTH, 9:00 a.m. - 5:00 p.m. (EST). E-mail address: docdelivery@haworthpress.com].

STATEMENT OF THE PROBLEM/CHALLENGE

An important guide for social work educators in implementing the use of information technology (IT) in social work curricula is how information technology is currently being utilized by social work practitioners in human services agencies. A better understanding of that utilization context should influence how we educate and train practitioners to function in that environment. Although the technological and information-based revolution has already begun, Helprin (1996) and others argue that it has not been developed with any sort of discipline or with any direct benefit to the people it should serve. First the science sector, then the business sector, and now the human services sector have adopted these technologies, but often without a clear sense of purpose. The benefit of automating some routine tasks in the business sector has proven itself repeatedly. However, the more complex tasks typical of the human services and social work have not fared as well (Schoech, 1995). Compared to its potential, full utilization of IT in the human services–and in social work education–appears to be lagging (Seaberg, 2001; Raymond & Pike, 1997; Butterfield, 1995) despite the possibilities it holds for improving the provision of human services (Schoech, 1995). A better understanding of why information technology has not fared as well as it should has direct implications for social work educators. This paper examines factors associated with underutilization of IT and offers a theoretically-based direction for future curriculum development.

Literature from the human services focusing on the issue of introducing information technology is reviewed, as well as literature from the business sector and the social sciences, to provide a broader perspective on the challenges posed by innovation diffusion. Next, Rogers' (1995) innovation diffusion theoretical framework is presented to promote a deeper understanding of how diffusions spread. This examination is selectively contextualized within the ongoing values debate in social work (Reamer, 1993). Combined, this analysis has direct implications for the social work education curriculum and future research.

REVIEW OF THE UTILIZATION OF INFORMATION TECHNOLOGY IN THE HUMAN SERVICES

In an early effort to assess the utilization of information technology in the human services workplace, Frans (1989) surveyed a systematic random sample of the entire membership of NASW. Over 54% of his sample (N = 520) utilized information technology for word processing and accessing client data in a database, but decision support and e-mail were used less than 5% of the time, and automated client assessment only 6% of the time. Only 10% of the respondents were involved in adopting a particular system, and only 22% were even consulted about system development. Only 52.6% had received any computer training, and of the total sample of 520, only 15 had received any type of undergraduate or graduate training in the use of electronic communications.

Other early attempts to understand the utilization, or lack of utilization, of information technology in the human services workplace are characterized by an author who asserted that since most frontline social workers were women and since social workers primarily work with persons of lower socioeconomic status, the current [1989] limited usage of information technology in social work reflected a combination of disinterested, less technically-oriented women and non-demanding clients (Cnaan, 1989). Such a conclusion today would be viewed as gender- and class-biased; nonetheless, it represented a view that was held by some in the field at that time.

Mutschler and Hoefer (1990) investigated diffusion issues from a process perspective, from the line worker through middle management, to uncover those factors that contributed to its underutilization. Their research indicated that structured tasks in human service organizations were the easiest to automate, but that automating unstructured tasks, such as decision support and outcome evaluation, would take more time. However, and most importantly, they found that attitudes toward information technology did not determine usage, a point we will return to later in the discussion.

Semke and Nurius (1991) noted the "poor fit" between technological innovations in the human services and the internal organizational environment. The authors specifically addressed "practitioner resistance" to information technology utilization and analyzed it in terms of the differences between micro and macro practitioners. However, their interpretation of the literature indicates that they perceived evaluation and measurement as key in the "development and implementation of automated information systems" (p. 355). This perspective on conceptualizing information technology has had a long and far-reaching impact upon the way most social workers view information technology in the workplace.

While some authors were looking at organizational issues affecting information technology usage, others continued to examine intrinsic worker issues affecting the lack of utilization. One such study was conducted by Monnickendam and Eaglstein (1993), who surveyed a sample of agency-based human services workers to find a set of descriptors or variables that could predict a worker's frustration with using information technology in the workplace. Some of these variables were hypothesized to be worker's sex, age, and amount of experience with information technology among other variables. What they found, however, was that neither age, gender nor lack of prior experience seemed to have any lasting effects on perceived attitudes towards computers once workers started using them in their daily routines. Frustrations with information technology, as such, were limited to lack of training and reliability/access problems related to any particular application. Overall, the impact of information technology in the workplace was modulated by "organizational and system design issues" over any "intrinsic attitudes towards computer utilization."

Several information technology and human services conferences have been held since the 1980s, with a primary observation being that the utilization of information technology in the human services has lagged far behind its potential capabilities. Some conference participants noted that the literature regarding information technology in the human services had largely been dominated by those contributors from the "rationalist perspective" and as such had largely focused on improving "organizational rationality and efficiency" (Geiss & Viswanathan, 1986, p. xxi). Furthermore, the political and value aspects of information technology had not received commensurate attention.

A more recent conference, the Information Management in Social Services Conference held at the University of Bath in 1995, was convened in response to growing awareness that information technology had refocused the need for "managers" to develop effective strategies to handle new stores of information. The conference proceedings discussed information technology utilization from a traditional, managerial approach, with no mention made of other uses or users (Kerslake & Gould, 1996). An exception was discussion of a newly emerging innovation in information technology, the Worldwide Web (WWW). Interestingly, it was felt the general public would not use the WWW in the foreseeable future because the cost would be too high; therefore, it would remain largely in the hands of those in the professional domains.

In summary, the literature demonstrates that a number of efforts have been made to understand the utilization of information technology in the human services workplace, and its underutilization, and recommendations have been made to expand its future usage. However, the determinants of utilization remain poorly understood. Moreover, the literature is largely atheoretical; and most attempts at conceptualization have taken place from a positivist/rationalist perspective. This paper will now examine utilization issues from a broader philosophical base and apply innovation diffusion theory to better understand this evolving process.

INNOVATION DIFFUSION THEORY

Perhaps the person most synonymous with innovation diffusion theory is the social scientist Everett Rogers, whose work on the topic dates back to 1962. Rogers defines an innovation as "an idea, practice, or object that is perceived as new by an individual or other unit of adoption" [e.g., an organization] (1995, p. 11). Diffusion is "the process by which an innovation is communicated through certain channels over time among the members of a social system" (p. 5). Innovations share the following characteristics that affect how quickly they will be diffused: (1) *Relative advantage*–the degree to which an innovation is perceived as better than the idea it supersedes; (2) *Compatibility*–the degree to which an innovation is perceived as being consistent with the existing values, past experiences, and needs of potential adopters; (3) *Complexity*–the degree to which an innovation is perceived as difficult to understand and use; (4) *Trialability*–the degree to which an innovation may be experimented with on a limited basis; (5) *Observability*–the degree to which the results of an innovation are visible to others.

While Rogers has contributed to the social science aspects of innovation diffusion theory, Abrahamson has contributed from the business perspective. Abrahamson (1991) challenged a seeming non-issue: that innovations diffuse when they benefit an organization and they disappear when they do not. He observed that not all good innovations diffuse, and more importantly, sometimes inefficient innovations diffuse even though they provide no benefit to the organization. He asserted that most organizational innovation diffusion theory has a pro-innovation bias which distorts the actual diffusion process for innovations.

This pro-innovation bias develops in situations when: (a) entities outside the organization, e.g., consultants, influence the choices made by the organization and when (b) organizations have unclear goals which make measuring technical efficiency difficult. For example, some organizations purchase information systems without undergoing a thoughtful and planned implementation process (TechSoup.org, 2000; Schoech, 1999).

Systems are purchased and implemented when no clear relationship has been made between the outputs of the system and the mission or goals of the agency. Abrahamson went on to outline 19 propositions that augment innovation diffusion theory. From these 19, this paper will address three that are particularly germane to this discussion.

Proposition 3 states that *inefficient innovations will diffuse when powerful groups back their diffusion* and Proposition 4 states that *technically efficient innovations will be rejected when powerful groups back their rejection.* These two propositions seem to typify the diffusion of information technology in the human services. On the one hand are the software applications that are implemented from the top down and which primarily serve the purposes of management without having any benefit to the direct services providers (Schoech, 1995). On the other hand are clinical assessment tools designed to improve efficiency in the assessment and delivery of treatment services that are underutilized by workers because they seemingly reflect a singular, empirical perspective. Proposition 13 focuses on the *diffusion aspect of "political costs" being weighed against "technical gains."* This proposition is supported by Rothman (1978), who believed that innovations are closely tied to influence mechanisms within an organization. The perceived net effect of an innovation is that some groups within an organization will increase in power and control, while others may diminish. This perception is only enhanced when an organization has unclear goals regarding its implementation.

Clearly, innovations do not diffuse in a haphazard fashion. The factors outlined above will either promote or inhibit the way any innovation will spread through an organization or, more broadly, through a profession. However, in addition to the technical aspects of innovation diffusion are the values aspects inherent to any innovation. Certain value and philosophical debates have been ongoing in social work for many years (Reamer, 1993). This debate, which has focused on the conflict between logical positivism (or empiricism) and heuristic positions on knowledge development (Reamer, 1993; Tyson, 1995), is closely aligned with Roger's discussion of the *compatibility* of values and needs, and also sheds light on why information technology has diffused so unevenly in our profession.

CONFLICTS IN SOCIAL WORK
CONCERNING VALUES AND NEEDS

The person who introduces technology into the human services workplace is typically a director or manager and, as such, occupies a position of authority and control over the workers, creating an unequal power balance. As long as the technological innovation is consistent with organizational goals and processes, the innovation should diffuse at an acceptable pace. However, when differences exist, the diffusion may spread slowly or not at all. The work routines of human services management, e.g., budgeting or accounting, are similar to those of the business sector and can readily be automated utilizing information technology. As noted by the previous authors, however, the tasks for the workers do not easily lend themselves to this automation. Therefore, the manifest benefit is more directly felt by management, while the workers are left working with a system that may not meet their needs. The fact that management now has a clearer advantage only serves to reinforce the power differential between the two groups.

Almost from the beginning, information technology in the human services came under attack from various authors for its dehumanizing effects upon the people who use it and the work they do. The two authors most associated with this cautionary note were Murphy and Pardeck (1991), who argued that left unchecked, computers represented the epitome of "rationalization" (p. 5), an artifact of logical positivism they felt excluded a more human influence. They based their argument on the basic component of computer information, the bit. As a binary unit, the bit can only have two values, 1 or 0, on or off; thus for information to be captured, it must be reduced to an either-or category and then codified. As an example, consider the marital status of a mother whose child has been reported to child protective services on two occasions. On the first occasion, she was married and on the second occasion, she was single. In the former case, her marital status might be interpreted as a potential asset, whereas her status in the second report might be screened as limited family support. However, additional contextual information might reveal that she was in a relationship marked by domestic violence at the time of the first report and on the second occasion she was single because she had left her abuser in order to protect her child.

Speaking more directly to the empiricist-heuristic conflict, LaMendola (1986) described social work's early dislike of computer technology as evidenced by the absence of any efforts in the beginning of the "information age" to develop software that was specifically suited to social work's needs and, in particular, its values. Instead, he asserted, we have spent many years importing software and applications from other professions, some of which have values that may conflict with social work's value base. Most importantly, software developers traditionally have focused on "intellect intensiveness or knowledge creation" [empiricism], whereas social work deals not only with knowledge creation, but also with the "beliefs, values, traditions, myths, and spirit of its clients and the world in which they live" (p. 7).

Of particular concern are the tensions between technologists who have a rationally- and empirically-based decision style versus practitioners, who utilize practice-wisdom and professional judgement (Krill, 1990). An illustration of this unintended consequence can be derived from a review of the software tools available for social work practice. Noting that social workers needed additional tools to further exploit the potential of the computer, Nurius and Hudson developed the Clinical Assessment System (CAS) program, which is a PC-based evaluation tool that allows workers and clients to assess client problems and monitor treatment progress over time. It utilizes an empirically-based single subject design that allows clinicians to conduct outcome evaluation studies (1988). An aggregate function is also built in so that an agency can examine its overall treatment effectiveness by program. In their later book (1993), Nurius and Hudson laudably attempt to cast a broader role for information technology in a human services agency; nevertheless, the overall tone of their work suggests an empirical/positivist perspective. While "networking" or communication is mentioned as a possible tool for the practitioner, the subject receives limited attention.

In another example, a program widely used in medical social work is MedSWIS (MedSWIS, 2001). It is primarily utilized to generate management reports pertaining to staffing and productivity, rather than clinical or case reports. The pro-management influence appears to be much the same in the non-profit sector. A cursory review of the software applications indexed at TechSoup.org (http://www.techsoup.org/) reveals that they primarily deal with administration, case management, financial management, fund raising, grants management, information and referral, membership management, outcomes management, planned giving, training software, and volunteer management.

IMPLICATIONS FOR SOCIAL WORK EDUCATION

Rogers' innovation diffusion theory offers an understanding of the limited utilization of information technology in the human services, and provides direction for social work educators seeking to increase utilization of IT in a way that is compatible with social work values and maximizes its potential. If social workers are to make full use of information technology tools in their workplace, one way to do so would be to learn how to use those tools during their formal social work education.

This education, however, needs to be guided by both innovation diffusion theory and our profession's values. In addition to straightforward instruction in how to use the computer, our schools can also model effective utilization behavior through various curricular activities. Applying Rogers' guidelines, implications for curriculum would include:

- Relative Advantage–Using the computer to access information highlights the greatest advantage IT has over other means of acquiring information. For the student, accessing an online database and retrieving articles is much more time-efficient than traveling to the library and trying to locate a journal that is oftentimes not there. This information acquisition process can then be transferred to the practice setting where accessing online community information may be more efficient than trying to keep track of numerous paper directories or service guides.
- *Compatibility*–This is the one issue that has had perhaps the most decisive influence on how IT has diffused in our profession. While the social work literature suggests that the positivist tradition has dominated the IT discussion, alternative perspectives suggest steps that can be taken to broaden IT's appeal. These steps should include:

1. Utilize applications that capture the communicative and collaborative aspects of professional social work practice, such as e-mail, listservs, and chat rooms. Gilbert (2001) argues that the full potential of e-mail in the non-profit context has yet to be realized. Instructors can model the use of e-mail through class listservs, reviewing drafts of papers via e-mail, or simply corresponding to students regarding learning activities outside of the predefined classroom hours. Assigning group projects where students communicate with eachother and the instructor will illustrate the potential of e-mail in facilitating collaborative efforts. Establishing guidelines for such usage would assist social workers once they are in the field and encounter clients or colleagues who choose to utilize e-mail to augment any face-to-face meetings.
2. While the positivist epistemological perspective is also implicitly communicated to social work students by the almost exclusive instruction in the use of SPSS (Statistical Package for the Social Sciences) or SAS (Statistical Analysis System) in research methods

courses, qualitative research approaches are now being discussed in introductory research texts (Rubin & Babbie, 2000; Grinnell, 1997). However, little has changed since Lindsey's (1977) discussion of SPSS and SAS as the primary tools to use in data analysis. While qualitative data analysis tools are available (Drisko, 1998), students who want to learn how to use these tools, e.g., NUDIST, NVivo, or Ethnograph, are typically referred to Sociology or Anthropology departments on campus, if at all. Instead we should educate our students to use these qualitative data analysis tools by using social work datasets to answer social work research questions.

3. *Complexity* as a barrier to IT utilization has continued to decrease as the user friendliness of the computer has increased. Nevertheless, providing students with hands-on time in the classroom will help dispel many misconceptions or fears about the difficulties associated with the use of technology. Furthermore, social work educators should make use of the computer in the classroom, as well, to model this behavior.

4. *Trialability*–Related to complexity is the issue of trialability. Our profession has only partially heeded LaMendola's (1986) warning that social work has to rely on others to design software applications for our own purposes. As such, we have had to make do with applications designed by those with a possibly different values base and user perspective, Nurius' and Hudson's (1993) contribution notwithstanding. The process of re-customizing an application can be expensive, so any feedback from trialability efforts goes largely unheeded. However, schools of social work can be used as test beds for new human services applications. Management classes would be the ideal setting to trial administrative applications; direct practice courses to trial new clinical applications; and community practice courses the natural setting for testing group or collaborative practice applications.

5. *Observability*–If the above objectives are achieved, then *observability* should be served as well. That is, students as imminent practitioners will be able to see the benefits of IT as a useful tool in the arsenal of skills they will bring to their professional practice.

Finally, Rogers makes particular note regarding the role of the *communicator of the innovation*. In social work education, this status and power is typically attributed to the professor. Therefore, unless specific precautions are taken, IT may become associated with the status and domain of the educational setting and not transferred to the social work practice setting. Therefore, the following recommendations should be followed:

- Introduce information technology as a bridge between the roles of social work student and social work practitioner. To wit, the utilization of IT as a teaching tool can serve to facilitate the transition from social work "student," who, in large part, may be dependent upon an educational institution for a particular phase in her or his life in order to gain the skills necessary to enter the profession of social work, to a social work "knowledge worker" (Wickramasinghe & Ginzberg, 2001), that person who is now an independent practitioner and capable of assuming many of the tasks necessary to continue the development of her or his professional skills. While the former implies an unequal power balance between the school and the student, the latter conveys a message of a collaborative partner in a power-sharing environment.
- Make use of databases and knowledge resources publicly available over the **WWW**. For example, much of our current graduate social work education introduces students to online journals or advanced statistical tools that may be unavailable to them once they graduate. The implied message is one of dependency upon the institution of higher education in order to develop continued professional skills. A different message would be conveyed if students were introduced to tools, either calculative, informational, communicative or collaborative, that were freely available via the **WWW** and that would allow them as practitioners to continue their professional development autonomously, no longer unnecessarily dependent upon the university.

IMPLICATION FOR FUTURE RESEARCH

The university setting provides a natural environment to research *trialability* issues in developing new social work IT applications. Rather than soliciting social workers' feedback after an application has already been developed, input should occur at the beginning of the conceptualization process, with specific attention being given to Rogers' frameworks. That is, applications should be conceptualized within the context of epistemology (both positivistic and heuristic) overlaid with compatibility, complexity, observability, and trialability features. Prototypes could then be developed, evaluated, and modified as needed. Schools of social work would not have to do this research alone. Many universities also have on their campuses either computer science departments or business departments with computer science programs that can facilitate some of the technical requirements. Such collaborative partnerships could leverage the best skills from both social work and the computer sciences as social work students, along with their professors, conceptualize applications that meet the needs of our profession, ranging from direct practice, through community practice, human services management, research/evaluation, and policy analysis. Rogers' theory should result in applications that better serve our profession and enhance the services provided to our clients.

Our society, and indeed the world, is most likely ushering in the Information Age during this millennia. In and of itself this event will be neither inherently good nor bad. The difference will lie with the way social work addresses this Age with the tools, values, and beliefs that have brought our profession to where we are now. The recommendations presented here do not require advanced knowledge of information technology; but rather, appreciation of our social work values as the foundation for the use of technology in the future of the profession.

REFERENCES

Abrahamson, E. (1991). Managerial fads and fashions: The diffusion and rejection of innovation. *Academy of Management Review, 16*(3), 586-612.

Berg, M. (1998). The politics of technology: On bringing social theory in technological design. *Science Technology & Human Values, 23*(4), 456-490.

Butterfield, W. (1995). Computer utilization. In R. Edwards (Ed.), *Encyclopedia of social work* (Vol. 1, pp. 594-613). Washington, DC: NASW Press.

Butterfield, W., & Schoech, R. (1997). The Internet: Accessing the world of information. In R. Edwards (Ed.), *Encyclopedia of social work* (1997 supplement, pp. 151-168). Washington, DC: NASW Press.

Cnaan, R. (1989). Introduction: Social work practice and information technology–An unestablished link. *Computers in Human Services, 5*(1/2), 1-15.

Drisko, J. (1998). Using qualitative data analysis software. *Computers in Human Services, 15*(1), 1-19.

Frans, D. (1989). *The diffusion of information technology and social worker empowerment.* Ann Arbor, MI: University Microfilms International.

Geiss, G., & Viswanathan, N. (Eds.) (1986). *The human edge: Information technology and helping people.* New York: The Haworth Press, Inc.

Gilbert, M. (2001). The Gilbert e-mail manifesto (GEM). Retrieved November 26, 2001, from the World Wide Web: http://news.gilbert.org/gem

Grinnell, R. (1997). *Social work research and evaluation: Quantitative and qualitative approaches.* Itasca, IL: F.E. Peacock.

Helprin, M. (1996, December 2). The acceleration of tranquility. *Forbes* (ASAP Supplement),14-22.

Hudson, C. (2000). At the edge of chaos: A new paradigm for social work? *Journal of Social Work Education, 36*(2), 215-230.

Kerslake, A., & Gould, N. (Eds.) (1996). *Information management in social services.* Brookfield, VT: Ashgate.

Krill, D. (1990). *Practice wisdom: A guide for helping professionals.* New York: Sage.

LaMendola, W. (1986). Software development in the U.S.A. *Computer Applications in Social Work and Allied Professions, 3*(1), 2-7.

Lindsey, D. (1977). General purpose computer packages in the social sciences. *Social Work Research and Abstracts, 13*(4), 38-42.

MedSWIS Software (2001). Retrieved November 26, 2001, from the World Wide Web: http://www.medswis.com/

Monnickendam, M., & Eaglstein, A. (1993). Computer acceptance by social workers: Some unexpected research findings. *Computers in Human Services, 9*(3/4), 409-424.

Murphy, J., & Pardeck, J. (1989). Technology, computerization, and the conceptualization of service delivery. *Computers in Human Services, 5*(1/2), 197-211.

Murphy, J., & Pardeck, J. (1991). *The computerization of human service agencies: A critical appraisal.* Westport, CT: Auburn House.

Mutschler, E., & Hoefer, R. (1990). Factors affecting the use of computer technology in human service organizations. *Administration in Social Work 14*(1), 87-101.

Nurius, P., & Hudson, W. (1988). Computer-based practice: Future dream or current technology. *Social Work, 33*(4), 357-362.

Nurius, P., & Hudson, W. (1993). *Human services practice, evaluation, and computers: A practical guide for today and beyond.* Pacific Grove, CA: Brooks/Cole.

Pasmore, W. (1988). *Designing effective organizations: The sociotechnical systems perspective.* New York: John Wiley & Sons.

Raymond, F., & Pike, C. (1997). Social work education: Electronic technologies. In R. Edwards (Ed.), *Encyclopedia of social work* (1997 supplement, pp. 281-299). Washington, DC: NASW Press.

Reamer, F. (1993). *The philosophical foundations of social work.* New York: Columbia University Press.

Rogers, E. (1995). *Diffusion of innovations* (4th ed.). New York: Free Press.

Rothman, J. (1978). *Fostering participation and promoting innovation: Handbook for human service professionals.* Itasca, IL: F.E. Peacock.

Rubin, A., & Babbie, E. (2000). *Research methods in social work.* Belmont, CA: Brooks Cole.

Schoech, R. (1999). *Human services technology: Understanding, designing, and implementing computer and Internet applications in the social services.* New York: The Haworth Press, Inc.

Schoech, R. (1995). Information systems. In R. Edwards (Ed.), *Encyclopedia of social work* (Vol. 2, pp. 1470-1479). Washington, DC: NASW Press.

Seaberg, J. (2001). Use of the Internet and other teaching tools in graduate social work education: A national survey. Retrieved November 27, 2001, from the World Wide Web: http://www.people.vcu.edu/~jseaberg/teaching_survey.htm

Semke, J., & Nurius, P. (1991). Information structure, information technology, and the human services organizational environment. *Social Work, 36*(4), 353-358.

TechSoup.org (2000, April 29). The planning process: Write the plan. Retrieved from: http://www.techsoup.org/articles.cfm?topicid=11&topic=Technology%20Planning

Tyson, K. (1995). *New foundations for scientific social and behavioral research: The heuristic paradigm.* Boston, MA: Allyn and Bacon.

Wickramasinghe, N., & Ginzberg, N. (2001). Integrating knowledge workers and the organization: the role of IT. *International Journal of Health Care Quality Assurance, 14*(6), 245-253.

Index

T - #0523 - 101024 - C0 - 212/152/13 - PB - 9780789029621 - Gloss Lamination